LAP-BAND
For Life

by

Ariel Ortiz Lagardère,
M.D., F.A.C.S.

Dedication

I wish to dedicate this book to those listed here. They have inspired and motivated me to pursue Weight Loss Surgery as a way of life and giving.

My wife Cynthia, the love of my life, for putting up with me either in the operating room or for so many sleepless hours at the computer writing this book

My newborn baby Alexa, you are an undreamable dream come true.

My Family, thank you Mom and Dad for giving me a chance at my realization

My Mentors, especially Mitiku Belachew, you are the man behind a dream that has come true for so many; thank you for inspiring me to follow in your footsteps

To all those patients who dared to hope and for all the incredible faith, intense love, and courageous strength you have shown to realize your dream; a dream has become a lighter, better healthier you— a Lap-Band for life.

The Author

Acknowledgments

I wish to thank the following individuals and groups for their collaboration and support in writing and completing this book. With this combined wealth of knowledge, our goal of providing an up-to-date and complete book on the LAP-BAND has become a reality.

- **Mitiku Belachew, MD** is not only the inventor of the LAP-BAND System, but also the first surgeon ever to place a LAP-BAND in Sept of 1993. He lives and practices surgery in Huy, Belgium. He is also my mentor and spiritual godfather.

- **Lee Grossbard, MD** has one of the most successful LAP-BAND practices in the United States. He is considered one of the top experts and travels frequently proctoring other surgeons and as an invited speaker to LAP-BAND seminars around the US. He is also a personal friend and admirable example to follow.

- **Franco Favretti, MD** is a pioneer in Gastric banding. He paved the way for the success of the LAP-BAND around the world. He practices at the Obesity Center of the University of Padua, Italy.

- **Roberto Rumbaut, MD** is another famous name from Mexico. He is the leader in LAP-BANDing in Mexico and is a band patient himself. He is credited with teaching numerous surgeons, worldwide, the technique and enjoys one of the busiest LAP-BAND centers in Monterrey, Mexico.

- **John Dixon, MD** has been with the LAP-BAND since the beginning, and is the author of numerous studies on the benefits of the LAP-BAND. He is credited with scientifically proving all the major health benefits and advantages of the LAP-BAND surgery.

- **Jeff Allen, M.D.** who is the Assistant Director for the Center for Advanced Surgical Technologies at Norton Healthcare/University of Louisville Hospital, Louisville, Kentucky

- **Jaime Ponce, MD,** also a Latin name, who is an outstanding leader in LAP-BAND surgery in the United States. He has developed a number of techniques and instruments and travels around the North America proctoring other surgeons. In addition, he has a very successful practice in Dalton, Georgia.

- **Terry Simpson, MD,** author of the book, *Weight-loss Surgery, a Lighter Look at a Heavy Subject*, is also a recognized weight-loss surgeon in his field. He is one of the handful of surgeons that perform the Biliopancreatic Diversion in the United States.

- **Arturo Martinez, MD,** a Bariatric Surgeon who has designed and implemented a number of safety protocols and surgical techniques related to LAP-BAND surgery. He practices with me at Obesity Control Center in Tijuana and Cancun, Mexico.

- **Gabriela Miranda, M.D.** has several degrees in medicine and nutrition. She is a medical doctor at the Universidad Autonoma de Baja California as well as having a Fellowship in clinical nutrition from the

Universidad Autonoma de Baja California, plus a Master's Degree in nutrition.

- **Velma Moreno Bandy** is president of V&V enterprises and is considered an expert in the field of reimbursement and insurance coverage for the LAP-BAND.

- **Bart Bandy** is the Senior Vice President of Field Operations for Inamed Health. He worked on a global basis for the company prior to leading out in the introduction of the LAP-BAND System in the United States. His commitment to quality, professional education and the development of a dedicated organization has resulted in the creation a leading medical device company. His passion for providing this safer, more efficacious procedure to more patients and surgeons is shared by every member of the Inamed Health team.

- **Vern Vincent** shares the credit for promoting the LAP-BAND's use. He has traveled extensively around the world, teaching others the techniques of the LAP-BAND and continues to actively work on innovations at Inamed Health.

- **Sandy Johnston** is a successful LAP-BAND patient and today actively assists others to reach their weight-loss goals. She has proven to have amazing insight on the way we think about food and losing weight.

- **My Patients.** Most of all, I would like to thank all of my patients who provide me with a feeling of fulfillment that I cannot describe. Each one of them has taught me and my staff how to help others succeed with the Lap-Band, and it is thanks to them that we have completed this book. I truly have the most wonderful people in the world as patients and I feel a personal connection to each of them. I would especially like to thank those that courageously shared their stories in this book in order to help others who suffer from this disease: Cynthia Jones, Dr. Lee Grossbard, Gayle Muller, Rick Rush, Carolyn Williamson, Shanae Scott, Teresa Quinoa, Lisa Geraci-Rupert, Dan Lester, Sandy Johnston, and Cassie Divello. We can all say we have the "LAP-BAND for LIFE"!

Ariel Ortiz Lagardère, M.D., F.A.C.S.

Table of Contents

Foreword

The first human laparoscopic gastric banding (LAP-BAND) for the treatment of morbid obesity was performed in September, 1993. We performed animal lab experimental work prior to 1993. The object was to define a surgical technique of laparoscopic approach in the obese patients. A considerable number of band prototypes were devised and tested before the standard LAP-BAND® could be completed.

The advantages of laparoscopic surgery as compared with conventional surgery were well known in the early 1990s. At that time the laparoscopic explosion occurred and allowed for a less traumatic experience with surgeries, among them was the laparoscopic cholecystectomy. It was considered a contraindication and a surgical challenge in severely obese patients due to a deep and difficult surgical field where there was massive visceral fat, hypertrophic and steatosic liver, as well as inadequate instrumentation. On the other hand, the possibility of performing bariatric surgery by laparoscopy offered a minimally invasive surgery on morbidly obese patients usually considered at high risk.

The main challenge surrounded the need to overcome technical difficulties in regards to laparoscopy in the morbidly obese. It was mandatory to have the advantages of laparoscopy without compromising the efficacy of gastroplasty, in regard to weight loss without acceptance of a higher rate of morbidity and/or mortality that would have been comparable to open procedures. In fine, it was not to be forgotten that the minimally invasive nature of the laparoscopic procedure in no way could be exempted from the obligation for a multidisciplinary approach to patient selection. This involved pre- and post-operative patient care and devoted follow-up, guaranteeing good results and good quality of life. This is the reason mastery of advanced laparoscopic technique, while compulsory, was not sufficient to undertake laparoscopic surgery in the morbidly obese patients. It was essential that extensive experience in morbid obesity management in general and conventional bariatric surgery be adhered to.

After the first human LAP-BAND operation, 25 consecutive patients underwent LAGB in a clinical trial program. This trial set of procedures was undertaken in order to define the feasibility, safety and efficacy of the procedure as applied in humans.

We held our first International Workshop on Laparoscopic Adjustable Silicone Banding (LASGB) at the Centre Hospitalier Hutois, Huy, Belgium. Thirty surgeons from around the world took part in this first workshop. They performed live operations with complete interaction with the participants. Training sessions in animal lab workshops gave the surgeons the opportunity to learn and familiarize themselves with the technique. By June 1994, the LAP-BAND became available to be used by trained surgeons.

After the first workshop, additional LAP-BAND workshops were organized in many parts of the world. One of those locations was Mexico City where the author of this book, Dr. Ariel Ortiz trained. He learned the procedure rapidly and achieved such great success with patients that I offered him the position as an outstanding instructor to train other surgeons, principally in North America. He was that skilled.

The introduction of LAGB (Laparoscopic Adjustable Gastric banding) in bariatric surgery has become a considerable breakthrough. Besides its total reversibility and adjustability understood in conventional bariatric surgery, it introduced the notion of minimal invasiveness. It is not by mere chance that the laparoscopic band gave a new boon to bariatric surgery in general and the laparoscopic approach in particular for the treatment of morbid obesity.

Obviously the LAP-BAND is not a panacea in obesity surgery. It is well known that weight loss after a restrictive procedure such as banding is sometimes less than the malabsorptive procedures. Nevertheless, as confirmed by its outstanding spread and extensive use since its emergence, laparoscopic banding deserves a preponderant place in the surgical treatment of morbid obesity for its undeniable qualities described above.

The development of LAGB has come about through a team effort that has united clinicians and engineers in a scientific spirit. The experimental work from a research concept attained the achievement of clinical application of a project without bending the rules of medical ethics. It is my belief that the introduction of the LAP-BAND in bariatric surgery has been more than a breakthrough; it has been, without doubt, a paradigm shift.

Eleven years after the first LAP-BAND surgery on humans, and hundreds of thousands procedures in the world, a comprehensive layman's book needed to be written. *LAP-BAND for Life* by Dr. Ortiz fills that gap. It is well documented, complete and above all, timely.

Mitiku Belachew, MD

Introduction

The history of weight-loss surgery is one of continuing evolution in search of safer procedures and of more effective permanent weight-loss results. I believe that adjustable gastric banding by a wide margin is the safest and most effective way to achieve permanent weight-loss for the severely obese. This book was written to fill a need for information on this surgery and attendant lifestyle changes, primarily for three groups:

- Obese and overweight people considering weight-loss surgery.
- Friends and relatives of the above group.
- Healthcare professionals who need to enhance their knowledge of the LAP-BAND procedures, its advantages and disadvantages compared to other procedures, and also to understand the aftercare that is involved.

Not everyone will want to read every chapter. For example, Chapter 6 on the medical details of the LAP-BAND procedure will be of importance to the healthcare professionals at which it is directed, of interest to people considering the operation, and not that important for friends and relatives. Here is what we consider to be the importance of the various chapters for each group:

Application of Each Chapter

* General Knowledge   **** Important**   ***** Vital**

CHAPTER NUMBER	CHAPTER NAME	GROUP I	GROUP II	GROUP III
		PATIENT	FAMILY & LOVED ONES	HEALTH CARE PROVIDERS
1	The LAP-BAND	**	**	***
2	Development of the LAP-BAND	*	*	***
3	Beware...FAT KILLS	***	***	***
4	The Workup	***	**	***
5	Selecting a Surgeon	***	**	**
6	Performing the Surgery	***	**	***
7	After the Operation	***	**	***
8	Fills—Getting the Band Adjusted	***	*	***
9	Guidelines and Nutrition for Success	***	**	***
10	Hunger, Pains in the Brains	**	**	**
11	Insurance Reimbursement	***	*	**
12	LAP-BAND over Bypass	*	*	**
13	LAP-BAND for Adolescents	*	*	**
14	Life after the LAP-BAND	***	*	**
15	Troubleshooting the Band	***	*	***
16	FAQ about the Band	***	**	**
17	Their Success Stories	**	**	**

What Can the LAP-BAND Offer You?

The following chapters discuss the subject in natural progression. There are three major sections of this book, divided into chapters, that discuss the LAP-BAND and how it came to be; the surgery itself and what to expect; and living with the LAP-BAND after surgery. Other interesting chapters address issues on how to decide where to get the procedure, how to finance it, etc. We will also discuss new and exciting applications being developed as we speak.

This book is dedicated to future patients thinking of having the procedure. Also patients who have undergone the procedure will benefit from it. If you are not a patient but are willing to further your knowledge on the subject to support a loved one's decision, this is the book for you. Last, but not least, healthcare professionals will also benefit from the information discussed in each chapter.

Terminology Note

The term LAP-BAND is used generically throughout this book to refer to the physical device and the surgical procedure used to implant an adjustable gastric band. Properly, LAP-BAND® should refer to the Inamed BioEnterics LAP-BAND System®, which is currently the only band approved by the FDA. Soft bands such as the MIDBand® and the Swedish Band® have been used for years outside the United States, and many Americans have them. The regimens are identical for these bands and the Inamed product, and are therefore referred to in the book with the generic term LAP-BAND®.

Words of Wisdom

Sound Advice:

Medicine is a blessing to all those who need it. For those who provide it, it is a never-ending, up-to-date science, while never losing focus of the compassion that must be involved in performing it. I have written this book from all the knowledge and wisdom I have amassed during this decade of experience from other experts as well as my own. The only truth I know is that which has already occurred (evidence based medicine) and can only foresee the future as an educated guess. Medicine is ever-changing as life itself.

As patients you are obligated to follow the wisdom of your surgeon as much as humanly possible. This guide is meant to be an inspiration to do just that. Every surgeon I have ever met in the world has only one goal in mind: to perform a perfect surgery that completely cures or controls a disease and either saves or provides a better quality of life while doing so. We are not gods; we are his servants, doing his work. Please, when in doubt, consult your surgeon.

Ariel Ortiz Lagardère, MD FACS

1

The LAP-BAND

Contribution by Dr. Franco Favretti

The LAP-BAND device is an implantable silicone ring designed to be placed surgically around the top of the stomach, with the ability to adjust it as long as it remains in the body. This concept, though not new, is unique in that it prevents overeating and fullness reached with less food, thus causing weight loss. This makes the LAP-BAND procedure truly an advantage over any other weight-loss surgery currently available.

An expert said that the LAP-BAND is revolutionary. This is true when you realize that the procedure eliminates stapling that is prevalent in some weight-loss surgeries. Not only is it less invasive, but it is also adjustable for each individual patient. The fact that the LAP-BAND is placed laparo-scopically through tiny incisions that are each less than 2 cm allows for a rapid 24-hour recovery in most patients.

The LAP-BAND Adjustable Gastric Banding System is an innovative and patient-preferred surgical approach to treating the significant and widespread medical problem of obesity. It provides surgeons and patients with a minimally-invasive intervention designed to help severely or morbidly obese patients lose weight. The procedure is adjustable and reversible, and does not require cutting or stapling of the stomach or gastrointestinal re-routing to bypass normal diges-tion. Patient benefits include a reduction in surgical trauma, complications, pain, and scarring, as well as shorter hospitali-zation and recovery times as compared to alternate obesity surgeries.

Severe obesity is a degenerative and debilitating dis-ease. The National Institute of Health reports that obesity substantially raises the risk of morbidity and mortality from:

- Coronary Artery Disease
- Diabetes
- Stroke
- Hypertension
- Sleep Apnea
- Cancer
- Respiratory Problems
- Osteoarthritis

Obesity kills more than 300,000 Americans every year, according to many institutional and governmental sources that will be detailed further on. Nearly everyone knows that losing excess body weight drastically reduces health risks. For example, 95% of patients with Type 2 (adult onset) diabetics who lose most of their excess weight no longer have diabetes. Doctor Paul O'Brien and his colleagues in Australia studied over 1,000 LAP-BAND patients and determined that major diseases such as high blood pressure, diabetes, sleep apnea, and asthma were controlled or resolved 90% of the time with the loss of excess fat. This is astounding.

This substantial increase in health risks has made obesity the second leading cause of preventable death in the United States. According to the American Obesity Association, obese individuals have a 50–100% increased risk of death as compared to normal-weight individuals, with 300,000 to 587,000 deaths each year. Because many people who lose weight by dieting regain the weight, surgical procedures have evolved to help morbidly obese people improve their chances of permanent weight loss. The American Obesity Association states that obesity-related costs exceed $200 billion per year in the United States.

The Ideal Weight-loss Procedure

Half a decade has been spent perfecting weight-loss surgery techniques. This decade alone has seen the use of laparoscopic (keyhole) surgery to make these techniques even more patient-friendly. What do we seek in the ideal weight-loss procedure? For one, it has to be effective. This means you should lose at least 50% of your excess weight. It also has to be safe. And though there are inherent risks involved in having surgery, especially in obese patients, complication rates should be low. Furthermore, it should be ideal in that it does not require stapling or re-routing of the intestines. It should not cause vitamin deficiency or malnourishment. Adjustability would be desirable, since our bodies are ever changing, and last but not least, it should be reversible.

This amazing method of dealing with weight control is the most outstanding feature of the revolutionary concept of weight-loss surgery tools. The LAP-BAND is safe and effective like no other weight-loss surgery currently available today.

The band is manufactured by INAMED BioEnterics LAP-BAND System®, referred to for simplicity in the rest of these pages as the LAP-BAND.

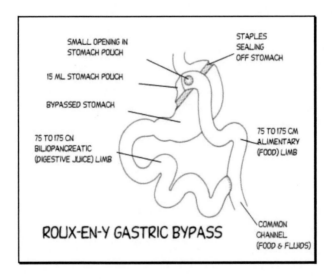

The Roux-en-Y Gastric Bypass

Up to now, the most popular weight-loss procedure in the United States is the Gastric Bypass, also known as Roux-en-Y and RNY. The term "stomach stapling" is a misused popular term for the operation, but other procedures include stapling of portions of the stomach, such as the VBG or Vertical Banded Gastroplasty. Following is a diagram of the Roux-en-Y Bypass procedure.

The popularity of the Gastric Bypass is due to a number of factors. For one, it has been used for weight loss for a couple of decades and was first performed laparoscopically in the United States. Weight-loss is much faster initially, and this has also contributed to its popularity. More health insurance providers will also cover the cost of having the Gastric Bypass.

The New Trend

The LAP-BAND was developed in Europe and spread to Australia and Mexico. There it was perfected, and only then were surgeons in the U.S. trained to perform it. I should know; I trained many of my colleagues in the U.S.

So why is the LAP-BAND not as popular as the Gastric Bypass? Because of a visionary and strict protocol. The manufacturer of the LAP-BAND requires a surgeon to assist in a two-day workshop, headed originally by international experts from Europe, Australia, or Mexico. Then they receive hands-on experience, performing the surgical procedure under the supervision of one of these experts, which is known as a proctoring. Only then can a surgeon apply the LAP-BAND for clinical use. This process has been slow, but many major centers and hospitals around the U.S. now offer the LAP-BAND.

Another reason it took a while to catch on was due to bad outcomes, complications, and poor weight-loss experienced early on during the FDA trials in the U.S. As surgeons became more experienced, results were promising and now are similar to those reported around the rest of the world.

New studies are now reporting that the LAP-BAND is not only safer than any other procedure, it is also as effective as the Gastric Bypass. This new insight will further increase the popularity of the LAP-BAND and is further discussed in the following paragraphs.

In a recent poll, obesity surgeons were asked what surgery they would choose to have performed on themselves or a loved one. The overwhelming majority chose the LAP-BAND!

Safety of the LAP-BAND

Unfortunately, when deciding on weight-loss surgery, most patients are only familiar with the Gastric Bypass surgery and not the LAP-BAND. And though patient awareness is on the rise, much work is still needed to properly inform patients of their options. The findings in studies indicate that the risk of death following the Gastric Bypass procedure is 1 out of 200 and that it may truly be as high as 1 out of 50. This means that the risk of death from Gastric Bypass operations is very high compared to other methods of weight-loss surgery. Now don't get me wrong, the Gastric Bypass has passed the test of time as a proven surgical option, but there is a substantial risk involved in having this procedure performed, as the numbers demonstrate.

LAP-BAND surgery is ten times safer than any other effective weight-loss procedure.

Other factors that should be taken into consideration are the problems associated with vitamin deficiencies and malnutrition that are a constant threat to Gastric Bypass patients. This is due to malabsorption problems inherent in the operation. Following LAP-BAND surgery, malnutrition problems are quite rare.

The Comparison

Which is the better procedure? One recent study has analyzed over 100 scientific papers to determine the safety and effectiveness of the major surgical procedures available for weight loss and compared them for safety and weight loss.

The surgical options were compared.

- Diet, Drugs, and Exercise Only (non-surgical)
- Gastric Bypass Procedure (GBP)
- Vertical Banded Gastroplasty (VBG) or stomach stapling
- Adjustable Gastric Band (AGB) LAP-BAND

At the start, all three groups of obese individuals had a number of health problems (co-morbidities) related to obesity such as Type 2 diabetes and the health problems it causes: degenerative joint disease, hypertension, coronary artery disease, gallbladder disease, certain types of cancer, gastroesophageal reflux disease (GERD), sleep apnea, asthma, psychological problems such as depression, greater risk during pregnancy, etc.

Of the *Diet, Drugs, and Exercise Only* group, these conservative options to attempt to control obesity have had ineffective results. A small percentage lost their excess weight, but as a group, their obesity-related health problems multiplied, and a significant number have died or will die from related illnesses.

Of the *Gastric Bypass Procedure (GBP)* group, the short-term mortality rate is 0.50%, but one reputable study indicated that nearly 2% died within 30 days of the surgery. The overall complication rate for this type of surgery was 23.6%, meaning that nearly 1 out of 4 will experience a complication with this Gastric Bypass Procedure.

The *Vertical Banded Gastroplasty* (VBG) group had a mortality rate of 0.31%, which proved a little less than the previous group, while patients undergoing this type of stomach stapling had an overall complication rate of 25.7%, even higher than the previous group.

The *Adjustable Gastric Band* (AGB) group had an overall mortality rate of 0.05%. This was drastically lower than the mortality rates mentioned for the previous procedures, with an overall complication rate of 11.3%, half of what is reported for the other surgical options.

The LAP-BAND is the winner!

After analyzing all the major studies reported in the world on weight-loss surgery, these are the facts:

- LAP-BAND is ten times safer than the Gastric Bypass.
- The Gastric Bypass results in more weight loss up to two years after surgery.
- Two to Four years after the procedure there is no difference in weight loss between the Gastric Bypass and the LAP-BAND.

When less is fine, more is not necessarily better.
The LAP-BAND offers a safer surgery with fewer complications, but it also proves to be a milder, more patient-friendly method of weight loss. These recent findings support the premise that with weight loss being equal at two years, why would one choose to have the riskier, more invasive operation?

After reading all this hard data, we vote for the LAP-BAND as the safest surgical method and with equal weight loss as the more popular procedure.

Because of its safety, we have also ventured into new applications, including its safety and effectiveness in adolescents. It has also proven to be effective in rescuing failed Gastric Bypass and stapling, and in offering a second chance to those who regained their weight.

FACT: Having the LAP-BAND procedure is safer than any current weight-loss surgery and clearly safer than doing nothing at all.

As you can see, there are several options to performing weight-loss surgery, however, the safest and most often performed throughout the world is the LAP-BAND procedure. It is not only the safest surgical procedure for weight-loss surgery, but it may also offer the best overall results.

Interview with Dr. Franco Favretti:

Q: Dr. Favretti, would you describe how the LAP-BAND has dramatically changed the way surgeons currently perform weight-loss surgery?

A: Dramatic innovations have occurred in the surgical field, mainly in the 90s. Among these innovations is the advent of laparoscopic or keyhole surgery that has had a real impact on the everyday surgical activity.

Behind the achievements of laparoscopic surgery and its related advantages, there is a new philosophy that requires an up-to-date risk and benefit analysis, plus a new respect for the anatomical and functional integrity of the patient; in other words, the patient's quality of life becomes the most important issue.

Laparoscopic Gastric Banding (the LAP-BAND System) is one of the procedures that most complies with this new surgical approach, and it is one of the best examples of "functional" surgery.

Q. As pioneers in this field, what is your insight on how this surgery has replaced other more invasive and complex procedures that are not functional?

A. The LAP-BAND fully addresses the need for a milder and more functional surgery that will provide the patient with weight loss without being extreme or radical. The LAP-BAND is truly a provider of "quality of life."

Dr. Favretti works at the Vicenza Regional Hospital in Vicenza, Italy, as well as the Obesity Center of the University of Padua. He developed and standardized the surgical technique for the laparoscopic application of Gastric Banding with Dr. Guy-Bernard Cadiere in September, 1993. The technique has been adopted worldwide by most surgeons employing the LAP-BAND.

2

Development of the LAP-BAND
Chapter by Dr. Mitiku Belachew

It all started in the early 1990s as a challenge: Could we develop a safe, effective, *and laparoscopic* surgical procedure for the treatment of morbid obesity? Here, in detail, is the rise to challenge that led to the development of the LAP-BAND® Adjustable Gastric Banding System.

The advent of laparoscopy, the marvelous surgical innovation that allowed for much less trauma in surgery by making small incisions, inserting a camera and instruments to maneuver about, and cutting and suturing, is a great boon to banding. It was a dream come true. Sometimes they refer to the surgery as *keyhole surgery*. This revolutionized the way surgery could be performed. The potential benefits to the patient were many: less pain, faster recovery, smaller scars, and less overall trauma, to name only a few. Though this new technique was extremely promising, the procedure was also technically demanding, so the prospect of performing this type of surgery on morbidly obese patients in a deep operative field, massive visceral fat, hypertrophic and steatotic liver, combined with inadequate instrumentation, created a particularly daunting challenge.

Still, we knew that if the problems could be solved, the advantages of laparoscopic abdominal surgery would be spectacular for these obese patients in whom conventional (laparotomic) surgery was known to be associated with increased risk of morbidity and mortality. If this new technique could be mastered, we could make a minimally-invasive procedure available to these patients who are usually considered high risk for open surgery simply because of their obesity.

The task was to conquer the technical difficulties of this new technique and to maximize its advantages without compromising weight-loss efficacy and without having to accept a higher rate of morbidity or mortality.

Before we could undertake the project of laparoscopic bariatric surgery, we had three problems to consider:

1. **Type of Operation:** When we began considering a laparoscopic gastric restriction operation, we possessed mastery of open Vertical Banded Gastroplasty (VBG) and open Adjustable Silicone Gastric Banding (ASGB). Thus, we needed to determine which of the two would be most appropriate to use in laparoscopy. We decided that the

gastric band, in addition to its other advantages, would be the less difficult gastric restrictive operation to perform laparoscopically, while still guaranteeing the qualities of the gastroplasty. Banding of the stomach for weight loss was not a new concept. In 1986, Lubomyr Kuzmak developed a silicone band with an inflatable (adjustable) balloon for the treatment of morbid obesity in his institution in New Jersey. His operation had many advantages: it was less invasive to the stomach; it was adjustable and, when necessary, reversible.

2. **How does one overcome the technical difficulties** of laparoscopic surgery in a fatty surrounding, coupled with a deep operative field, with the hypertrophic liver and bulky omentum? How could one avoid the risk of perforating the posterior wall of the stomach? Furthermore, was there a need for special instrumentation for laparoscopic bariatric surgery, notably extra-long trocars and dissectors (the surgical tools that would need to be inserted through the tiny incisions)? So, at the beginning of the project we understood the necessity of establishing a new protocol for laparoscopic surgery applicable to severe obesity.

3. **The existing silicone band** of Kuzmak was not readily adaptable to laparoscopy. Thus, new prototypes of a silicone band for laparoscopic use needed to be designed, fabricated, and tested. For ethical reasons, the experimental work was to be performed in an animal lab to allow the development of the laparoscopic surgical technique for obese patients and to define pitfalls, complications,

and feasibility without too much risk. Concurrently, prototypes of laparoscopic silicone bands were tried.

The Dream

Development began in 1991, when Dr. Belachew submitted a plan for a research program for the development of a laparoscopic surgical technique for the laparoscopic placement of a band. The transcript of our proposal in the records of the BioEnterics Corporation (manufacturer of the ASGB) included a two-stage research program: an animal model to be performed on pigs and a human model once all initial trials were performed.

Phase I - The Animal Model (a pig)

This phase allowed for the development of the laparoscopic surgical technique with mastery of all the dissection problems and the creation of a silicone band adapted for laparoscopic use.

Phase II - The Human Model

This phase was dependent on Phase I and conditioned by two questions: (1) Could the operation be performed safely? and (2) Was the laparoscopic silicone band created? The application of the procedure in humans could not be undertaken without the approval of the project by an ethics committee and acceptance by the patients after informed consent.

Once these prerequisite conditions were met, clinical trials could start with voluntary and consenting patients. To evaluate feasibility, safety, and efficacy, 25 consecutive operations would be performed. After that, international workshops would be organized to teach the technique to surgeons.

Questions to Answer

First, we needed to determine the size of the band. Then the question is asked, was the band to be attached to the stomach by suturing? Could we imagine a self-locking mechanism? Was it necessary to add reinforcing sutures in addition to the locking mechanism? Was placing the band laparoscopically feasible? What were the possible complications? What would be the causes of these complications, and how could they be avoided? There were a myriad of questions to be answered. While we were working in the animal lab on the project, some surgeons started laparoscopic operations using other types of bands directly on humans in 1992. Dr. Catona in Italy performed laparoscopic placement of vicryl and silastic bands. The gastric pouch had a 50 ml capacity and a stoma diameter of 12 to 15 mm.

Dr. Cadiere in Belgium laparoscopically inserted the first generation ASGB (designed for open surgery) in a female patient. Concurrently, we proceeded with the evolution of a sequence of ten prototypes of the silicone band during the experimental phase in the animal lab.

The result was the development of a self-locking band, diameter adjustable by inflation or deflation with saline solution, and designed to be placed laparoscopically.

Next, the development of a standard laparoscopic banding technique, an operation with maximum safety:

- Description of all the steps of the procedure from initial dissection site to end of operation.
- Definition of feasibility conditions, difficulties, and pitfalls.

In June 1993, a video of the Laparoscopic Adjustable Gastric Band in pigs was presented at the Annual Meeting of the American Society for Bariatric Surgery (ASBS). This presentation was greeted with great enthusiasm and our first operation in humans was anticipated with interest.

The Reality

We were fully satisfied with Phase I of the experimental work (Animal Model). We submitted a protocol for its application in humans to the Ethics Committee of the Centre Hospitalier Hutois, Huy, Belgium, and the Committee unanimously approved the project.

We then performed the first human Laparoscopic Adjustable Gastric Banding on September 1, 1993, at the Centre Hospitalier Hutois, Huy, Belgium. The procedure lasted three hours and there were no intra- or post-operative complications. The patient has had excellent long-term weight loss, and currently is regularly followed and feels satisfied.

From September 1993 to February 1994, twenty-five consecutive patients underwent Laparoscopic Adjustable Gastric Banding in the clinical trial program as the operative techniques were refined. The clinical trial was intentionally initiated on female patients with gynoid obesity and BMI 40–45 kg/M2. Later, patients with a greater BMI were included in the surgical testing.

A series of bands, with lengths of 9.5 to 13 cm, were initially manufactured. For the clinical trial, however, only two sizes (9.75 and 10 cm) were maintained, as they could cover all the requirements if the dissection protocol was strictly respected.

In March 1994, the First International Workshop on Laparoscopic Adjustable Gastric Banding was organized at the Centre Hospitalier Hutois, Huy, Belgium. Thirty surgeons from around the world took part in this first workshop. Live operations that included complete interaction with the participants were performed. Training sessions in the animal lab during the workshop gave the participants the opportunity to learn the technique, and there was widespread enthusiasm. Later, workshops were organized in other areas of the world.

No Sales of the LAP-BAND to Surgeons without Training at an Approved Center.

The policy of the LAP-BAND's manufacturer (INAMED Corporation, Santa Barbara, California, formerly BioEnterics Corporation in Carpinteria, California, USA) was not to sell the device to surgeons until they had participated in a training program at an approved center. The required surgical experience before surgeons were admitted into a training program included acceptable experience in bariatric surgery and advanced laparoscopic skill, e.g., laparoscopic anti-reflux surgery. Experience and qualifications in the management of obese patients were also necessary, as the surgeon's first duty was to do no harm to the patient.

More than ten workshops were held in our center, and we trained more than three hundred surgeons. At the end of each workshop, special recommendations were given to the trained surgeons to insure that their first ten procedures would provide the best and most successful learning opportunity. These special recommendations were termed the TEN COMMANDMENTS OF LAP-BAND SAFETY.

In July 1994, the LAP-BAND System became available on the international market for use by trained surgeons. In June 1995, the Food and Drug Administration (FDA) approved the start of clinical trials in selected centers in the United States. FDA regulations require clinical trials in approved centers before an implantable device (such as the LAP-BAND) can be used in a surgical procedure. Dr. Belachew was involved in proctoring all of the surgeons in these trials. Six years later, the FDA approval of the LAP-BAND System in the U.S. was granted on June 5, 2001. Meanwhile, the LAP-BAND had been extensively used in many countries since 1994. It is estimated that more than 140,000 LAP-BANDs have been implanted worldwide at this writing.

Although the initial LAP-BAND System model has needed very little modification since its first use in 1993, the technique of its placement has required significant change due to late complications. These complications were related essentially to enlargement of the gastric pouch due to pouch dilatation, per se, or stomach slippage. Many patients with pouch dilatation/stomach slippage required a second surgery. Although revision surgery could be performed by laparoscopy in 80% of patients (band repositioning or band removal), the high rate of these complications (more than 10%) was not acceptable.

The reason for this complication was analyzed. After a learning period, we found that pouch dilatation and/or stomach slippage was caused by creating too large of a pouch. The anterior wall was also partially mobile due to insufficient suturing. Another cause was the stoma becoming too tight due to postoperative edema.

Beginning in 1995, we changed the surgical technique in order to prevent pouch-related complications, and we now believe that the pouch-related problems have been at least partially solved by these modifications of the technique.

Review

The introduction of Laparoscopic Adjustable Gastric Banding to bariatric surgery has been a considerable breakthrough. Besides its adjustability and reversibility, it introduced the notion of minimal invasiveness. The laparoscopic band created a growing acceptance worldwide in bariatric surgery, in general, and the laparoscopic approach, in particular, for the treatment of morbid obesity.

The development of the LAP-BAND has been the result of teamwork that united clinicians and an engineer in the scientific pursuit. The experimental work achieved clinical application following the rules of medical ethics. The dream became a reality.

Author:

Historically, only a few talented people around the world have been able to reach out and touch hundreds of thousands of people to give the gift of life. Dr. Belachew, the author of this chapter, is one of those brilliant surgeons who have achieved that lofty status.

3

Beware...Fat Kills!
Contribution by Dr. John Dixon

Just what does obesity mean to you? Obesity is simply excessive storage of fat in the body. It is fat you don't need. Body fat can be measured to determine the amount that is present in the body, and from those measurements it is possible to distinguish what is normal and what is not for a particular body structure.

One of the first methods to determine body fat and arrive at an acceptable ideal weight was a method designed by Metropolitan Life Insurance in the 1980's. Unfortunately, this table did not take into account the weight and height differences between ethnicities and countries. Today a better measurement for obesity is the current method known as the *Body Mass Index*, or BMI.

The BMI formula is an individual's weight in kilograms divided by the square of their height in meters. The formula is fairly simple. You divide your weight in pounds by 2.2 in order to equate kilograms. Multiply your height in inches by 0.0254 to arrive at meters. Also, you can go on the Internet and calculate with easy-to-follow instructions by typing in the search engine BMI calculations. This method is a good measuring tool for just about anyone except extremely muscular people such as bodybuilders who may weigh in as high on the BMI scale, but in reality have little excess fat.

BODY MASS INDEX KEY		
BMI	CLASSIFICATION	LEVEL OF HEALTH RISK
Under 18.5	Underweight *	Minimal
18.5 - 24.9	Normal Weight	MInimal
25 - 29.9	Overweight	Increased
30 - 34.9	Obese	High
35 - 39.9	Severely Obese	Very High
40 and over	Morbidly Obese	Extremely High

This table is from Standards Committee, American Society of Obesity Surgery; Obesity Surgery.

Currently, there is an even more accurate way of measuring body fat to determine whether you have excess weight. This is done by means of a body fat analysis that includes a mechanical and electronic method of measuring body fat. This popular technique is a procedure where a very low voltage current is passed though the body and measures total body fat. It is likely that in the future the scientific community will concentrate more on this method of measuring fat than other methods because it yields such accurate results. And who knows, perhaps one day a much more improved means of measuring will be devised.

There are those who have asked if obesity is due to a hormonal problem or an eating disorder. Doctors estimate that hormonal imbalance is to blame for excess fat in less than 2% of the morbidly obese patients. They also estimate that less than 2% of the morbidly obese have an eating disorder.

Today, we now understand that obesity in almost all cases is a disease and this refutes the usual explanation for obesity as a lack of willpower. Furthermore, studies indicate that less than 2% of obese people are able to permanently go from being overweight to normal through willpower alone. In other words, it doesn't work for them.

In 1998, former U.S. Surgeon General Dr. C. Everett Koop stated that obesity is "the second leading cause of preventable death in the United States." Smoking is the first. Dr. Koop and two noted authorities on obesity, JoAnn E. Manson, M.D., a professor at Harvard Medical School and Theodore B. Van Itallie, M.D., Professor Emeritus of Medicine at Columbia University, gleaning data from the 1995 Federal Centers for Disease Control and Prevention (CDC), noted that 1.6 million deaths in the United States were from "natural causes." What is interesting and alarming is that over 300,000 of those deaths were attributable to excess weight. What is more, most of those deaths were preventable and would not have occurred if the people who died had lost their excess weight.

This was a report in 1997. What will the data reveal now? It could be of epidemic proportions. Other researchers put estimates of deaths due to obesity from 300,000 to over 500,000 per year. And in addition, obesity increases the risk of illness in about 30 serious medical conditions. For example, an obese person is 6 times more likely to develop gallbladder disease and 6 times more likely to develop high blood pressure that leads to strokes and Alzheimer's disease.

Being 10% overweight raises the risk of a heart attack by 30%, especially if the extra pounds are around the belly. Obese people develop heart disease seven years earlier than those who remain thin. Also, obese people typically register high levels of HDL (bad) cholesterol and triglycerides. Then, too, there are those among the obese who struggle with diabetes. The obese are 3.8 times more likely to develop diabetes. Medical researchers estimate that between 88% and 97% of the cases of Type 2 (adult-onset) diabetes that have been diagnosed are obese patients. There is a five-fold increased risk in those who are moderately overweight and a ten-fold increased risk in those who are severely obese.

Over 20 million Americans have Type 2 diabetes that we now know is obesity related. What is even more startling is that more than a third of them do not know they are diabetic. This is an ailment that is the leading cause of blindness, kidney failure, amputations, and heart disease.

The American Diabetes Association says obesity, combined with a genetic predisposition, increases the risk for the most common form of diabetes, called Type 2. The percentage of adults in the United States with Type 2 diabetes is as follows:

- **Underweight** (BMI under 18.5): 4.7% men; 4.8% women
- **Normal weight** (BMI 18.5 to 24.9): 2% men; 2.4% women
- **Overweight** (BMI 25 to 29.9): 4.9% men; 7.1% women
- **Obese class 1** (BMI 30 to 34.9): 10.1% men; 7.2% women
- **Obese class 2** (BMI 35 to 39.9): 12.3% men; 13.2% women
- **Obese class 3** (BMI 40 or over) 10.7% men; 19.9% women

Australian researchers report that the BioEnterics® LAP-BAND® System surgery that limits the amount of food entering the stomach dramatically improved the health of seriously obese people with Type 2 diabetes.

The obese are twice as likely to develop osteoarthritis, plus they are subjected to higher rates of cancer. Cancer is increasingly linked to obesity, with the greatest number of those who have it suffering from prostate, cervix, and ovarian cancers. Overweight men have a 70% greater risk of colon cancer. A sixteen-year study of 900,000 people showed that obesity has contributed to 20% of cancer deaths in women and 14% in men. This amounts to a staggering figure of a 100,000 cancer deaths per year caused by obesity.

Medical Definitions of Obesity

Body Mass Index (BMI)=kg/m2		Medical Definition
Women	Men	
<17.5		Anorexia
<19.5	<20.7	Underweight
19.1-25.8	20.7-26.4	In Normal Range =Ideal Weight
25.8-27.3	26.4-27.8	Marginally Overweight
27.3-32.3	27.8-31.1	Overweight
>32.3	>31.1	Very Overweight or Obese
35-40		Severely Obese
40-50		Morbidly Obese
50-60		Super Obese

Obesity increases tremendously a woman's risk of getting breast cancer, and the likelihood of fatality; this is due to fat that makes it more difficult for early detection of tumors. Obesity keeps blood hormone levels high, making it harder to fight the disease. A new Yale study found that severely obese women are three times more likely to be diagnosed too late to fight the cancer. Then too, obese people have several times the incidence of bone and joint disease.

The US Center for Disease Control lists their findings of health issues related to obesity in the following order:

- High blood cholesterol, dyslipidemia
- Insulin resistance, glucose intolerance
- Hyperinsulinemia
- Angina pectoris
- Congestive heart failure
- Stroke
- Cholescystitis and cholelithiasis
- Gout
- Osteoarthritis
- Obstructive sleep apnea and respiratory problems
- Poor female reproductive health (such as menstrual irregularities, infertility, irregular ovulation)
- Uric acid nephrolithiasis
- Additional psychological disorders are prevalent; among these are eating disorders, distorted body image, and low self-esteem. Many obese people suffer discrimination in employment and academic situations.

There are social and economic factors to consider as well as illnesses. Overweight persons are far less likely to be hired than those who are thin. According to one study, the overweight people are often typecast as "emotionally impaired, socially handicapped, and possessing negative personality traits." Furthermore, wages for obese persons are lower by as much as 24% than those with acceptable weight levels.

Losing Weight Can Cure Diseases

Today we know that by losing weight we can lose or control diseases as well. For over 90% of patients who are successful in losing excess weight, diabetes, hypertension, asthma, sleep apnea, and a number of the other medical conditions mentioned above, gain control or even become cured. With this information concerning the effects of obesity as a health and economic hindrance, the question is asked, "What is being done and what will motivate weight reduction among the obese?"

Motivation

Younger people tend to be more motivated by appearance and self-esteem, while older people are often motivated by health issues. Other motivation factors include important events such as weddings, divorce, a new job, tight clothing, and the list goes on. Nearly everybody is contemplating weight-loss dreams of becoming thinner.

Health

Fear of obesity-related diseases rarely plays a role in the decisions of younger patients to lose weight. As patients age, however, the fears of developing diseases such as diabetes or hypertension appear to be a motivating factor.

Due to obesity-related diseases, the idea of drastic weight-loss becomes a major issue and many turn to weight-loss surgery to assist in the fight against obesity.

FACT: Obesity has now reached epidemic proportions around the world! It will probably be the major killer of this new millennium.

The Size of the Problem

Obesity in the United States has been on the increase for at least twenty years, according to an October 2002 article in *The Journal of the American Medical Association*, that was based on a U.S. government survey conducted in 1999 and 2000. Compared with a similar study by the government in 1988-1994, the percentage of American adults considered overweight increased from 56% to 64%, those considered obese increased from 23% to 30%, and those considered extremely or morbidly obese (BMI over 40) increased from 3% to nearly 5%. This constitutes a major increase in body weight.

Worldwide Estimates

Over the years, obesity levels have increased in all parts of the world in both industrialized and developing countries. We estimate conservatively that approximately 1% to 2% of the world's population is morbidly obese (BMI over 35, or more than 160% of ideal body weight calculated according to the 1983 Metropolitan Life Insurance Company tables). If those with mild and moderate levels of obesity are added (BMI from 25 to 35, or 120% to 160% of ideal body weight), this number expands by a factor of 17.

What about Diets?

Diets, pills, hypnosis, and exercise tend to be successful at assisting people in losing weight, but these regimens have several problems for permanent weight-loss. I have listed a few here:

- Only a small fraction of the people on diet programs persist for the years needed to lose their excess weight.
- Even those who persist lose only a small percent of their excess weight.
- The overwhelming majority who go on diets gain back most or all of the weight they lost on the regimen, and many become even heavier than before the diet.

Furthermore, only half of the subjects in a diet study of the four most popular diet regimens lost as much as 5% of their body weight. When compared to the norm of weight-loss for those who had LAP-BAND surgery, the success rate for LAP-BAND is much higher. The majority have lost 20% to 50% of their total body weight, and kept it off. Those who resort to other means of losing weight, such as Hypnosis, herbal treatments, and chemical supplements, have had even less success than those on various food diets.

Exercise works for a very small percentage of the morbidly obese of those who are able to persevere at an exercise regimen. However, the rate of weight-loss is so slow compared to weight-loss surgery that few can stay the course long enough to lose the 75% of excess weight common in LAP-BAND surgery.

FACT: Only permanent weight-loss leads to health benefits. Permanent weight-loss from dieting alone doesn't hack it.

Permanent weight loss from diets is far less than from Surgery. In a report on popular diets, there is interesting information for those who think these diets are really a solution to fighting their overweight battle. The report *One Year Effectiveness of the Atkins, Ornish, Weight Watchers, and Zone Diets in Decreasing Body Weight and Heart Disease Risk,* by Michael Dansinger, M.D. of Tufts-New England Medical Center, reported that his studies of 160 people who were divided into four groups of 40 had alarming results. The groups of overweight people agreed to follow each of four diets: Atkins™, The Zone™, Weight Watchers™, and the Ornish™ (low-fat vegetarian diet). The participants ranged in age from 22 to 72, and most were 30 to 80 pounds overweight.

According to Dr. Dansinger, maintaining the diets by the groups was not easy. He noted that after twelve months, 42% of the participants had stopped following the diet they were assigned. The drop-out rate for each diet was 22% at two months; by twelve months, half of the volunteers assigned to the Atkins™ or Ornish™ diets had dropped out, as had 35% of those assigned to the Weight Watchers™ or Zone™ diets. Of the remaining 58% who stuck to the diets, the average weight loss was 5% of their total body weight, regardless of the diet they followed.

This compares with average weight loss of 20% to 40% of total body weight for those who had undergone LAP-BAND or Gastric Bypass surgery, and it is interesting to note that only a very low percentage of surgery patients do not stick to the regimen that could result in significant weight loss.

Even with this relatively small weight loss of 5% of total body weight, those dieters who stuck to it reduced their heart disease risk by an average of 5% to 15%. Dansinger stated that losing 20 pounds corresponded to about a 30% reduction in heart risk score. He presented his results at a press conference on November 9, 2003, at the American Heart Association's Scientific Sessions 2003.

The extreme difficulty of diet and exercise as a means of weight loss is well documented. Gastrointestinal surgery, coupled with sensible food intake, along with exercise, is the best option for people who are severely obese and cannot lose weight by traditional means.

This lack of effective weight loss is the key reason that gastric LAP-BAND surgery is such a great tool for weight loss success. Keep in mind, however, that it is only a tool and you will have to do your part to make it effective; still in all, it is unique and doable as opposed to the wide array of diets and other remedies that are popping up everywhere.

Dr. Ortiz Interviews Dr. John Dixon:

Q: Dr. Dixon, how does weight loss affect major disease?
A: One of the most remarkable effects of weight loss following LAP-BAND surgery is the dramatic improvement or total resolution of disease associated with obesity. There are nu-

merous, common diseases strongly linked to obesity that are referred to as comorbidities of obesity. Type 2 diabetes is perhaps the best known and one of the most serious, where the link to obesity is so strong that the combined condition is often called *diabesity*. This progressive disease leads to deterioration in multiple organs and systems, and is the most common cause for adult blindness, limb amputations and renal failure in western countries, as well as the leading independent risk factor for coronary artery disease. If the disease is treated soon after diagnosis, and substantial weight loss is achieved, all clinical evidence of the disease disappears in the majority of patients. This is quite remarkable, as Type 2 diabetes was previously considered to be an incurable condition.

Q: What other common diseases may resolve with the LAP-BAND procedure?
A: Major improvements or resolution are seen with weight loss in other comorbid conditions that include high blood pressure, abnormal blood fats, obesity-related sleep problems, liver disease, breathlessness, infertility, and joint problems. These physical changes reduce the substantially increased risk of early death, especially death related to cardiovascular disease that is associated with severe obesity.

Q: Does the LAP-BAND and weight-loss affect mental health?
A: There are also major improvements in psychological problems suffered by the obese person. Body image, self esteem, self-confidence and mental health are all improved and there are fewer symptoms of depression. These positive changes in physical and mental health along with better exercise toler-

ance and mobility provide the background to greatly improved "quality of life" status. Patients, prior to surgery, report major impairment in all aspects of their quality of life; with weight-loss improvement so great that patients report quality of life measures identical to those of the general population. Few surgical procedures can provide such a broad, well-documented benefit to health.

4

The Workup

Contribution by Dr. Arturo Martinez

One of the most appealing aspects of LAP-BAND surgery is the safety with which it can be performed while dealing with people who are at a higher risk of having mild to life-threatening complications. It is because of this that all patients submitting themselves to gastric band surgery must have a complete medical evaluation that is independent of age, prior medical history, and current health status.

The evaluation is a team approach: it involves coordinators, a psychologist, nutritionist, cardiologist, and anesthesiologist, and of course, the surgeon. In some cases, when warranted, other medical specialties such as internal medicine, endocrinology, intensive care, and others are brought in.

The evaluation process starts by obtaining the patient's health history, which must also include a weight history. If that person meets selection criteria for surgery, then that person must undergo laboratory tests, chest x-ray, electrocardiogram, and pulmonary function testing (when warranted) before surgery. The patient is then evaluated by the different specialties involved. If no contraindication to perform the surgery arises, the patient is admitted to the hospital the same day of surgery and medications and measures are applied to diminish risks that may be involved, such as pulmonary embolism, infection, and acute heart and lung conditions, and to ensure a faster and more comfortable recovery. It is important to mention that because of the nature and safety of LAP-BAND surgery, it may play an important role in the treatment of morbid obesity in the pediatric adolescent population and people with resistant obesity with a BMI below 35.

PATIENT SELECTION CRITERIA FOR MORBID OBESITY SURGERY

- Body mass index (BMI) of 40 or higher
- BMI of 35 or higher with co-morbidities
- Long-term history of obesity with multiple unsuccessful attempts at weight loss (non-surgical)
- Ability to comply with dietary and behavioral changes as recommended by a weight-management team

Health History

It is important to obtain your health history as soon as possible during the entire evaluation process. Its scope is to detect any illness or situation referred to as a co-morbidity that can increase the patient's risk to surgery and at the same time know the state of control and problems related to that morbid state. This health history is usually obtained by questionaires. There are some illnesses that are of particular interest in patients that are to undergo surgery. Such illnesses are sleep-disordered breathing (sleep apnea), asthma, diabetes, high blood pressure, heart disease, deep-vein thrombosis, gastroesophageal reflux disease, and thyroid disease.

This health history must be obtained as early as feasible because modifications can be made that diminish certain risks (such as pulmonary complications) that can account for about one-quarter of all deaths occurring in the first six days after surgery. Also, prevention of heart-related problems and deep venous thrombosis (DVT) are of the highest importance.

Lowering Surgical Risks

Pulmonary Risk

You can do certain things to lower these risks. For example, stop smoking eight weeks before surgery has been proven to be very beneficial; even cessation of smoking two weeks prior to surgery has been proven to be of some benefit. Achieving the latter can be difficult for some, but it can be done by most people, especially if there is a sound understanding of what can be gained. Professional help and support groups are always a great tool for the patient when there is difficulty while trying to stop smoking prior to having surgery. If you are under treatment for any diseased condition, you must have the best control possible of the underlying illness in accordance with your primary care physician. In order to achieve this goal, a good doctor/patient relationship is helpful. In addition, doing some exercise such as walking or achieving some weight loss and having good medical control of any pulmonary illness, such as asthma, can have an impact on your outcome.

Pulmonary function tests are not done routinely on all patients since they haven't been proven to predict pulmonary complications in the postoperative period. But we will do them on any patient who has a background of pulmonary disease to determine if that patient is at that specific moment eligible for surgery. If the patient has a severe lung deficiency, he or she will be treated accordingly and prepared for surgery at a later date. Tests such as polysomnography (detects breathing abnormalities such as sleep apnea) are sometimes requested since most of the breathing abnormalities found in the morbid obesity patients are related or worsened by being overweight. Sleep apnea correlates with body mass index (BMI); the higher the BMI, the more probability of having this disorder.

It is not a contraindication for surgery, although sleep apnea with severe pulmonary restriction may be. These patients are best treated for weight loss by non-surgical means; even a small or moderate amount of weight loss can have a favorable impact on pulmonary function and make the procedure possible.

Heart Risk

Identifying risk factors for coronary heart disease is the key to prevention. Achieving good control of hypertension, diabetes, and serum lipids (cholesterol and triglycerides) is necessary for a good outcome. In some cases, this can be difficult because of the underlying problem of obesity, but it can be accomplished by most with proper treatment.

Physical activity and a modest weight-loss can have favorable effects on blood pressure and lipid and glucose metabolism before surgery. Most of the time, the role of identifying and treating risk factors falls to the skills of the primary care physician. For this reason, it is important to follow medical advice, take prescribed medications as ordered, and do your routine visits. Testing for heart disease (e.g., echocardiography, stress testing, catheterized, nuclear stress testing) is done based on clinical findings.

RISK FACTORS FOR CARDIOVASCULAR DISEASE	
Hypertension	Obesity
Diabetes mellitus	Sedentary
High blood cholesterol	Menopause
Smoking	Family history

Pulmonary Embolism (venous thrombo embolisim or VTE)

VTE refers to a condition in which blood clots are generated inside the venous vessels of the legs (deep venous thrombosis) and can ultimately travel inside the blood stream and wind up in the vessels of the lungs, causing mild to life-threatening situations and even death.

The incidence of VTE has gone down since more effective preventive measures have been developed and guidelines are developed, but it is still an important cause of death in hospitalized patients. The most important factors influencing the appearance of VTE are venous stasis, abnormal blood coagulation, and vessel endothelial damage.

The length of the operation is important because long-lasting procedures are associated with a higher incidence of VTE. In laparoscopic surgery, it is necessary to create a working space inside the abdomen by injecting a gas (CO_2), which in turn increases the abdominal pressure and favors venous stasis. In addition, placing the patient in a tilted position about 30 degrees with head up (anti-trendelemburg position) can also favor venous stasis. Immobility after surgery is also an important factor that can generate thrombosis.

This is why the experience of the surgical team is important; it is well known that most surgeons pass through a learning curve with surgical time reduced as experience grows.

All patients are treated with a "blood thinning" agent, usually a type of heparin, and compression stockings. Another type of device known as an intermittent pneumatic compression stocking is also used in high-risk patients. This device exerts intermittent pressure on the legs which leads to a good venous blood flow and avoids venous stasis.

In rare cases in which the patient has had a previous embolism while on adequate treatment or significant bleeding complications due to anticoagulation, the blood flow can be managed with a filter device that is placed in the inferior vena cava through a venous puncture and acts as a barrier for clots that can ultimately travel from the lower limbs to the lungs.

Bleeding

Because of the nature of laparoscopic LAP-BAND surgery, hemorrhage fortunately is a very rare complication. Patients who take non-steroidal anti-inflammatory drugs, such as aspirin, even in small doses on a regular basis, are asked to stop at least seven days prior to surgery since this type of medication is known to prolong bleeding episodes.

The LAP-BAND surgeon, in conjunction with the prescribing doctor, should determine when it is ideal to stop blood thinning agents. Oral anticoagulation agents such as Warfarin must be stopped 72 hours prior to surgery since they can prolong blood coagulation time and, therefore, hemorrhage. They are also difficult to control and counteract. Heparin and low-molecular-weight heparin are the substitutes of choice, and they are usually started the same day the oral anticoagulant is suspended and maintained 72 hours after. Oral medications are started within 24 hours of surgery for most patients. Other illnesses that can increase the chance of hemorrhage are usually a contraindication for this procedure (e.g., liver cirrhosis).

Infection

If any infection occurs prior to surgical procedure, it must be treated accordingly, for example, skin fungal infection which is common with large skin folds where humidity exists. Preventive antibiotics are usually applied in the hospital before the surgery to keep possibilities of infection in the wounds to a minimum and especially in the adjustment port area. Even though there is no bacterial contamination from viscera at the moment of the surgery, an infection can still occur owing to many factors which can be local (related to the wound) or generalized (systemic illness), for example, excessive dissection of tissues in the wound, fluid collections such as a hematoma (blood collection), or any illness that can affect host defenses. It is also worth mentioning that in the rare occurrence of an infection in any of the wounds, it is treatable with local drainage and antibiotic, and this rarely compromises the adjustment port or the band.

Avoidance of Other Risks

Although the chances of having any major complications are very rare and LAP-BAND placement is an overall safe procedure, you should not underestimate this possibility, because morbid obesity is synonymous with high risk. The relative risk for everyone is different. That is why it is important to be as accurate as possible when reviewing medical history, including past experiences with anesthesia and surgery, so that the medical and surgical team can take the preventive measures necessary to ensure a safe outcome.

Preoperative Diagnostic Workup

Medical History

Your medical history will aid us in distinguishing patients who are going to need additional testing or exams prior to the surgery. It is a very important tool for the clinician and must not be taken lightly. Special attention is given to co-morbidities (mentioned previously) with a detailed history of gastro-esophageal reflux disease (GERD) or any esophageal-related illness (since this may warrant specific studies and even a different surgical approach, such as the repair of a hiatal hernia commonly associated with GERD) and prior surgical and anesthesia experiences.

Diagnostic Testing
All patients are submitted to laboratory exams for a complete workup. Red and white blood cells, sugar, cholesterol, blood clotting, and urine are all tested. When deemed necessary, glycosylated hemoglobin is checked to assess glucose control. Added coagulating blood tests may be necessary for people on blood-thinning agents. If any abnormalities are found in the exams and corrective measures are needed, this is done prior to the surgery. An electrocardiogram and chest x-ray are performed frequently.

Endoscopy and manometry for esophageal reflux disease are done on an individual basis depending mainly on a history of GERD or surgery for hiatal hernia and GERD. They are also done routinely on patients with prior surgery of the stomach, such as Gastric Bypass or gastric stapling procedures.

Upper gastro-intestinal series (x-ray with oral contrast medium) is used in patients with large hiatal hernia or prior surgery, such as Gastric Bypass and gastric stapling. Its main purpose is to view the anatomy of the structures involved in the procedure and rule out any abnormalities that may cause difficulties or even contraindicate surgery.

Abdominal ultrasound testing is performed when symptoms related to gallstones are found. In the case of symptomatic gallbladder disease, it is best treated before surgery, or in some cases it can be done at the same time.

Physical Examination

Patients are evaluated by the cardiologist, surgeon, anesthesiologist, and other specialists when needed.

The physical examination must be thorough and done in an orderly fashion, starting from head to toes. Close attention is paid to detecting any signs of heart and lung disease. Attention is also paid to the oropharynx region, especially by the anesthesiologist since a short neck and large protruding tongue can predict difficult management of the airway and, therefore, the anesthesiologist can be prepared with all of the alternatives necessary to handle a difficult case.

Body Fat

Distribution of body fat, such as in apple-shaped obesity (compared to pear-shaped obesity), can predict a challenging surgery. Another factor that can make the surgery more difficult is a large-size liver. It is difficult to assess during physical examination, and is more frequently dealt with during surgery. Ultrasound can assess liver size, but it will not predict the difficulties a large liver can pose during surgery. This is why it is better to diet 7 days prior to surgery . . . you make it easy on the surgeons and also on yourself.

Other common findings are edema of the lower limbs and signs of venous insufficiency. It is important to know that special studies (like some already mentioned and other specialty consultations, although uncommon) are decided based on initial findings in the health history, test results, and physical examination. All of this is done to avoid any complications and ensure the safest procedure possible.

Day of the Surgery

Management before Hospital Admittance

Once you have completed the evaluation process and are approved for surgery—meaning that no contraindications were found—you will be admitted to the hospital and prepared for the operation. It is important to remind yourself to take essential personal items, especially when traveling a great distance. Make a checklist and include any questions you may have for medical and hospital staff. The following is an example of some things to take to the hospital.

PERSONAL ITEMS

- Recent or relevant medical records or test results
- Any medical device used by patients on a frequent basis (continuous positive airway pressure device or CPAP prosthesis of any kind)
- All essential medications (e.g., blood pressure and heart disease, diabetes, asthma, thyroid, other hormone replacement, pain killers, etc.)
- Personal hygiene items (e.g., Toothbrush)
- Other items such as reading glasses and reading material, comfortable clothing and footwear are optional

---

Please note that if the patient is taking medications that are essential for well-being, they will be continued prior to and after the surgery. We will mention some medications that are of importance:

- Antihypertensive drugs or other cardiovascular medications
- You will be asked to continue the medications even on the day of surgery. In some cases the patient is prescribed new medications or the dosage is modified prior to surgery to obtain better control of the underlying condition. Some people have no history of high blood pressure and experience hypertension before the surgery because of the generated stress; therefore, they will be prescribed medication to control such "stress" (usually a sedative) and, if necessary, medication for high blood pressure.
- Oral medications and insulin for diabetes
- These must not be taken on the day of surgery, and if the patient is insulin-dependent, it will be applied and controlled by hospital staff according to blood glucose levels, which are monitored carefully prior to, during, and after operation.
- Other types of drugs
  - o Thyroid and other essential hormonal-replacement medications can be taken on the day of surgery.
  - o Steroids are usually changed to an intravenous presentation.
  - o Migraine, allergy, and asthma medications can be given on the day of surgery if indicated after clinical evaluation.
  - o Remember to have a small amount of liquid with medications (¼ cup of water or less) and not to eat any food 8 hours prior to surgery.

Preoperative Treatment

Upon admittance to the hospital, the patient is asked to put on a hospital robe and remove all clothing and jewelry. Leg compression stockings and a peripheral intravenous catheter are placed. Medications are started:

- A blood-thinning agent is applied approximately sixty minutes before going to the operating room to diminish the risk of venous thromboembolism (VTE).

- Antibiotics (usually second- and third-generation cephalosporin or, in patients with a history of an adverse reaction to them, other types of antibiotics such as quinolones) are given to lower risk of skin port-site infection.

- Pre-anesthesia enhancers and sedatives are given by the anesthesiologist, clonidine, and lorazepam (benzodiazepine), respectively. They help to diminish the dosage of anesthetics given in postoperative pain control.

- Anti-nausea medication (Ondacentron or Zofran) is applied prior to surgery to all patients unless there is a history of intolerance to it, which is rare. The rationale for its use is that many people have adverse reactions (such as vomiting) to some medications, especially narcotic drugs, and it is impossible to predict who is going to have it. It is important to remember that the band is placed around the esophageal-gastric junction. This area is subjected to large pressure changes while vomiting, which can disrupt sutures or dislodge the band or stomach through the band (early slippage). This is why preventive measures are very important.

- Pain-control medication is sometimes started prior to surgical procedure; usually a non-steroidal anti-inflammatory agent is used (Parecoxib a COX-2 inhibitor).
- Antacid secretion medication is also started (Proton pump inhibitor) to protect gastric mucosa from stress and fasting.
- Inhaled bronchodilators are given to patients with a history of asthma or poor results on respiratory function testing.
- Other medications are used on an individual basis and as suggested by the evaluating medical team.

Once in the operating room, the patient is positioned on the surgical table and placed under general anesthesia. Care is taken to avoid unwanted time loss; even small ones that add up can prolong operating time and, therefore, cause complications.

Postoperative Hospital Care

After surgery, the patient will be monitored until fully awake from the anesthesia. This is usually a short period since most medications used are eliminated by the body within few minutes. You will be asked to walk as soon as possible; this can be achieved by most 1 to 4 hours after surgery, and you will be asked to walk frequently. All patients are started on breathing exercises every hour with a simple device called an incentive inspirometer, which has been proven effective in preventing pulmonary complications, and then if the patient is dependent on a CPAP (continuous positive airway pressure device), this procedure will be continued after surgery. Other therapeutic measures may be performed on an individual basis, depending on health status and surgical outcome.

POSTOPERATIVE ROUTINE

- Monitoring until fully awake.
- Intravenous medications and fluids are continued.
- Walk within 1 to 4 hours after surgery and continue walking frequently.
- Initiate breathing exercises once awake.
- Moisten mouth with ice chips once awake and initiate free intake of liquids 6 hours after surgery for most.
- Discharge, 9 out of every 10 patients within 24 hours after surgery.

Medications and intravenous liquids are continued for the next twelve to 24 hours. At this time most of the patients can be discharged from the hospital and told to continue their regular oral medications. In our experience, 90% of patients recover and are discharged from the hospital within 24 hours.

Summary
In bariatric surgery every effort should be made to ensure the safest procedure possible. This effort includes the patient and medical team together. A well-informed and motivated patient is always the ideal candidate for LAP-BAND surgery. Also, the experience, knowledge, and caring from everybody involved is key to success.

5

Selecting a surgeon

Eleven years have passed since the first LAP-BAND was placed. Back then a patient wanting to have the procedure had very few options—none in the United States. Now nearly 1,000 doctors have been trained in the technique in the US alone, and many centers have accumulated substantial experience.

There are three major deciding factors when selecting a LAP-BAND center or surgeon. One is experienced doctors and staff. Most international centers have performed thousands of LAP-BAND surgeries, but some centers in the US are quickly accumulating experience. So, maybe you will only consider the most experienced centers. Others look for convenience; if the center is just across the street, then that may be your first choice. Others consider the cost of the procedure if they are self-pay. This means they may have to travel to get to the center or surgeon they have selected. Some may look into all three—experience, convenience and price.

Here are described some important considerations when deciding where to have your LAP-BAND and with which surgeon.

Basis for Selection

When selecting a surgical team there are some things to consider. Do your homework on the surgeon who may be performing the surgery. Dr Flancbaum in his book *Doctors Guide to Weight-loss Surgery* considers three important things when deciding on a weight-loss surgeon: professional qualifications, experience, and personality (bedside manner). We consider this a very solid basis for selecting a surgeon. Other factors that may influence your decision will be where the surgeon performs surgery and possibly the cost.

Professional Qualifications

Surgeons in the United States

Bariatric surgery is becoming popular in the United States, and around the world for that matter. LAP-BAND surgery is becoming more accepted as patient awareness increases. All surgeons start from the beginning. This does not mean your surgeon will be less qualified to perform the surgery. It merely means they have performed fewer LAP-BAND procedures. Even so, this is not a good indicator of your surgeon's lack of proficiency. Other indicators such as the ones discussed below may be better indicators.

First, you want to know if your surgeon is board certified. This means that the surgeon has completed a general surgery program of at least five years and passed the examination administered by the American Board of Surgery. Check his affiliation with other medical societies related to general surgery or the practice of bariatric surgery. Fellowship in the American College of Surgeons is one of the most prestigious memberships a surgeon can have; this is usually designated by the initials FACS after MD.

Progressive surgeons tend to be active not only in performing surgery to their best abilities, but they are usually involved in evolution, innovation, and advancement of the medical sciences. They typically are also active members of bariatric societies such as *The American Society for Bariatric Surgery* or ASBS. Other important societies include IFSO or the *International Federation for the Surgery of Obesity.* (This is the granddaddy of all bariatric societies.) You can find the web links to these organizations in the appendix at the back of this book.

International Surgeons

If your surgeon is located outside the United States, all of the previous statements still apply as qualifications. Most countries have board certification for surgery. International surgeons can be *Fellows of the American College of Surgeons* (FACS) as well, and members of the *American Society for Bariatric Surgery* (ASBS). Frequently, they will be members of their local and regional societies. However, you should verify membership and affiliation from the organizations where they claim membership. An effective way to check on a surgeon is to contact the Regional or National College of Surgeons for their country or the IFSO International Federation for the Surgery of Obesity.

NOTE: Always check with www.INAMED.com (USA) or mecachrome-medical.com (Latin America) if you are not sure!

Experience

Will experience influence the outcome of a surgical procedure? Yes and no! While every surgeon has to start his or her experience on the first patient, most surgeons in the United States have an advantage. They have been trained by other international experts who have passed on vast experience and knowledge on the subject. Because of the strict protocol that the manufacturer of the LAP-BAND requires in order for a surgeon to perform a LAP-BAND, these approved surgeons are fully trained and proctored during their first cases, resulting in a rapid learning curve for the surgeon and a safe surgery for the patient. Each LAP-BAND surgeon is required to complete the INAMED training by an authorized proctor surgeon and have a proctor surgeon present during his or her first three surgeries. This proctor, I or another proctor surgeon, designated by INAMED, will ensure that the new LAP-BAND surgeon masters the proper surgical and placement techniques.

The United States is quickly catching up to the rest of the world. Many centers in the US have amassed a number of surgeries. The long-term experience is still dominated by international surgeons in Australia, Europe, and Mexico. What is the significance of this for a patient seeking a more experienced surgeon? A surgeon who has vast experience on the subject may resolve a complication or foresee it before it happens. It may also mean that the surgical time may be less and that their style of follow-up may be different or even more streamlined.

In our experience at our center, we have found that many patients will secure a doctor close to home for their follow-up care and fills. This is always a good idea and can come in handy when they are unable, for some reason, to return to our Center. Yet, often we see our patients back at our Center for follow-up care.

The reason for this is two fold. They have found that even with travel expenses, it is often more cost efficient to return to our Center. The second, and more common reason, is that many are having a difficult time obtaining a correct fill volume—known as the "sweet spot." The "sweet spot" refers to the patient comfortably eating approximately one-third of their pre-band amount of food without hunger and as a result successfully losing weight. We have found it to be beneficial to our patients to make every attempt to get them to their "sweet spot" quickly so that they can achieve maximum weight-loss in a least amount of time. In doing so, the patient's motivation remains high when they see a faster result.

Of course, it is impossible to predict with certainty exactly how many fills will be needed, but the average patient at our Center requires two fills the first year to achieve and maintain a correct fill level. We do, on occasion, have the rare patient that will require three or more fills the first year.

Band adjustments, like most things, become more accurate with experience. Some surgeons prefer to "sneak up" on the correct fill amount without using fluoroscopy guidance. There is no right or wrong fill technique; however, this technique is not usually used by international surgeons.

Wherever you decide to have your surgery, be confident that your surgeon is fully trained and supported to take on this surgery if his or her qualifications are in order. I have never witnessed such cooperation between surgeons as there is with those who perform the LAP-BAND procedure. We get numerous e-mails or phone calls at our Center from different surgeons asking questions about the procedure or follow-up. Societies like the ASBS have an e-mail-based support system that connects to all members.

The more experienced surgeons usually will emit their opinions on the subject. The LAP-BAND manufacturer also provides guidance for the surgeons who require further assistance or additional training. If your surgeon is performing the LAP-BAND, be confident that there is a vast network of experts supporting him and helping him in case it is needed. Technology is now helping us gain experience through communication.

Personality

This is a delicate matter and is personal to each patient. Surgeons are not all created equal. Often the things that matter are simple. Your surgeon should be willing to treat you with respect and compassion. He should take time to explain the LAP-BAND procedure, pros and cons, and answer all your questions. Bedside manner is important to most patients. Having surgery is never a pleasant event, so at least it should be uneventful and the surgeon reassuring. At the end of the day, these are the things that make your surgical experience less stressful and more relaxed.

If you don't feel comfortable with your surgeon and feel he or she is unapproachable, then you may be less likely to ask for assistance with your future questions and concerns. This could hinder your weight-loss success because follow-up is important for success with the LAP-BAND. You should also feel comfortable with the other professionals on the surgeon's team. They will most likely include at least one other surgeon, a nutritionist, psychologist, patient coordinator, and other staff members. You will be working with these professionals as well as your surgeon for possibly years to come. Make sure everyone on the team is courteous, respectful of you and your needs, and answers all of your questions. Don't let the staff move you along quickly. You should never feel rushed.

Ask the surgeon what his personal thoughts are concerning the LAP-BAND. Unfortunately, some surgeons still consider the gastric bypass the "gold standard" in weight-loss surgery. And while they will offer the LAP-BAND, they may attempt to dissuade you from LAP-BAND surgery by quoting old, outdated FDA trial results. Do you really want a surgeon to perform your LAP-BAND surgery if that surgeon does not believe it is a safe and effective treatment for obesity? Also, does he or she have all of the current data on the LAP-BAND and its effectiveness?

Convenience

Likely you may have to do a little traveling if you are selecting a surgeon based on experience, qualifications, and cost. Most major cities have at least one center offering this procedure. So, it does depend on what your priorities are.

If you live in an area where there is no surgeon currently performing the LAP-BAND, then regardless of whether or not you are self-pay or have insurance that will cover it, you will have to travel. Some will claim that you should always have surgery as close to home as possible in case there is a future complication. In a perfect world that would be true. However, the LAP-BAND is safer than any other weight-loss surgery and carries a low complication rate. It is very unlikely that you will have an emergency due to your LAP-BAND. Most of the time, a LAP-BAND emergency amounts to nothing more than the fill is too tight, which can be rectified by going to the nearest LAP-BAND surgeon available to remove some of the fluid. Not having an experienced LAP-BAND surgeon in your area should not deter you from getting a band placed. If you do travel for your surgery, do your homework and use our helpful guide on what to take. It will make your experience more pleasant.

Cost

If your insurer covers your surgical procedure and you are comfortable with the surgeons and surgical facilities they offer you, may still have to overcome obstacles that you may not have foreseen. Here are the major ones:

- Large amounts of qualifying questionnaires and forms
- A significant co-payment, often several thousand dollars
- A significant delay between starting the process and the operation, sometimes more than a year
- A limited number of surgeons to choose from

- Most American insurers cover only surgery in the United States with more stringent FDA requirements for qualifying than those used by surgeons in Europe, Australia, and Mexico. For example here are some issues that cause denial:
    o Patients with a BMI under 36 will automatically be denied
    o Patients with a BMI 36-40 must have significant co-morbidities (related illnesses)
    o Patients younger than 18 or over 60 may not be considered

Pay special attention if you have decided to travel to a foreign country for surgery. Most of these facilities offer a comprehensive information package, including all the travel information and support required to reach their center. I would caution against using price as your first priority for choosing a center, as less reputable centers will often cut corners in order to charge less than their competitors. No one should choose to accept less than the highest quality center to perform surgery. Surgery can and does affect your life!

Do your homework! If it sounds too good to be true, it usually is!

Self-Pay Patients

People who choose to pay for the surgery themselves fall into four groups:

- Those who have given up on the possibility that their insurer will cover their LAP-BAND surgery.
- Those whose insurers might cover the LAP-BAND surgery, but need or want the surgery much earlier than the red-tape-filled US insurers would allow.
- Those who are more comfortable being treated by the more experienced LAP-BAND surgeons who practice in Europe, Australia, and Mexico.
- Those who do not qualify under the American protocols.

Assuming you wish to self-pay, you next have to choose the surgeon you want to perform the operation. The first element of choice is location. As this book is being published in the United States, we will concentrate on typical options for North Americans.

In the best of all possible worlds, a laparoscopic surgeon with LAP-BAND experience would be nearby and would charge, with hospital fees, a reasonable amount. Again, if this is your case, go for it. It cannot get any better than this. For some North Americans, neither the price nor the surgeon will be ideal. The total charges in the US for surgeons, anesthesiologists, tests, and hospital are generally two to three times higher than those charged in Europe, Australia, or Mexico. Some US surgeons and medical centers are now offering packages where the total cost is only 50% higher than in Europe, Australia, or Mexico.

Even so, this option is usually limited to patients in a specific BMI range and is done on an outpatient basis, which reduces the costs incurred. If a patient's BMI is over a certain number, most US surgeons will require the procedure be done on an inpatient basis. This, of course, will be at a higher fee.

Some will not qualify even if they are self-pay. As I indicated above patients there may be restrictions with a BMI under 36, or patients with BMI 36-40, unless they have significant co-morbidities, or patients under 18 or older than 60. In such cases, patients have no other alternative than to travel outside the country to have a LAP-BAND placed.

If cost is a factor, be wary of Internet specials. Remember, you get what you pay for!

Where to Have Your Surgery

Most internet support groups are there to assist patients on their surgical weight-loss journey. There are some great support group message boards available. Some that have been suggested to me are: www.spotlighthealth.com and www.obesityhelp.com. These groups are broken down into subgroups for LAP-BAND and bypass patients. Also, there is www.lapbandtalk.com that offers excellent information. This group is also broken down into topics and geographical areas.

Our Center has also recently created its own support group board, www.lapbandforum.com. Everyone is welcome to join, and we encourage members to share stories. Then too, there is a LAP-BAND surgeon-locator service available at INAMED's website for American surgeons at www.inamed.com. There will also be an international surgeon locator on INAMED's Mexican LAP-BAND distributor web page, www.mecachrome-medical.com.

You will find other lists of domestic and international doctors on some of the Internet support groups and other places on the Internet. However, I highly recommend using the last two sites listed above that are the official sites of INAMED.

United States

Check out each surgeon who is in your region of the country. Find out the total cost of the package, how many LAP-BANDs the surgeon has placed, what kind of aftercare will be offered, and the cost of fills. Get a clear cost estimate and terms that the surgeon charges, plus and fluoroscopy charges. When you have narrowed your search down to two or three possibilities, contact the office staff for an initial consultation. Most established centers have support group meetings where you can meet other patients who have gone through the surgical experience with the doctor you are considering. You can also talk to other patients on line in specific chat groups, either dedicated to a certain doctor or by region.

Remember, a good source of information is the manufacturer of the LAP-BAND, INAMED Health. They are willing to talk to patients and guide them through the selection process.

If you are seeking LAP-BAND surgery outside the United States, the following options are available:

Europe

In Europe, there are a dozen or more surgeons who specialize in banding. Several have more than a decade of experience with banding. They place not only the INAMED BioEnterics LAP-BAND®, but also the MIDBand and the Swedish Band. Typical costs range from €6,500 to €11,500.

Some of the most famous LAP-BAND surgeons in the world practice in Europe. The leading countries are Belgium, Italy, France, and Germany.

Mexico

The more popular alternative for many Americans is choosing surgeons in Mexico because of proximity to the United States and thus the cost and convenience of travel is less expensive. There are LAP-BAND surgeons in Mexico City and throughout Mexico, but there are clusters of LAP-BAND surgeons in two key cities in Mexico: Monterrey and Tijuana. Each of these doctors, and the majority of their employees, speaks fluent English.

Monterrey

Monterrey is a modern industrial city with a population over a million, located about 300 miles south of San Antonio, Texas. Its hospitals are world class and the LAP-BAND surgeons there are among the best in the world, several of whom have placed more than 1,000 LAP-BANDs. Surgery in Monterrey typically costs approximately $10,000, which includes surgery, hospital charges, hotel charges for three days, and transfers to and from the airport. Fills have an additional charge when using fluoroscopy, which is usually in the $110 range.

Tijuana

Tijuana is an industrial and tourist city 15 miles from downtown San Diego, California. This hustle and bustle border town has a less than ideal reputation that it does not deserve. To the surprise of many, our center in Tijuana was selected by INAMED as a site for American surgeons to take their workshop courses that were hosted by Mexican and Australian surgeons. The surgeons in Tijuana are some of the best in the world, and the state-of-the-art facilities meet the same standards as the US. Tijuana has an edge over Monterrey due to cheaper and more frequent flights to San Diego. Currently, surgery in Tijuana typically costs $10,000, which includes surgery, hospital charges, and hotel charges for three days, and transfers to and from the San Diego airport. Fills are typically free for life, except for the cost of fluoroscopy, which is also in the $110 range.

Cancun

The name speaks for itself—paradise! Because of the international demand for LAP-BAND surgery, the authors have established a center in Cancun, reachable by commercial flight from practically any part of the world. Flights are available on a daily basis and are affordable. The package caters to world-class patients from every area of the globe. The complete experience includes a five-star hotel accommodation for five days, state-of-the-art surgical facilities, with transportation, meals, and other amenities all included. The cost is around $13,500. Currently this package is being offered by a top American surgeon from Florida teamed with the author. We felt that the need for quality care abroad for certain types of patients, such as those wanting to combine their surgery with a pleasant getaway, was clear, and we are happy to offer this option to provide patients with the opportunity for a healthy life.

Our future plans of expansion include Cabo San Lucas in Baja Mexico for West Coast patients.

Things to Remember If You Are Going Outside the US

Check the Surgeon and the Center

Most LAP-BAND surgeons who are internationally famous have built a reputation on the quality of their surgical abilities, combined with a state-of-the-art surgical center and a compassion for their patients. We cannot offer a lower price than that which has been quoted above without sacrificing quality and safety. Cutting corners is not recommended—ever. Once again, be wary of Internet specials and freebies. Surgery is a serious matter and it requires serious thought, especially if you are going to a foreign country. Complete your homework; investigate the surgeon's reputation; talk to some of the surgeon's patients. Many can be reached on chat groups.

Be aware that the laws governing advertising are not the same in other countries. This means is that some less reputable centers will make claims either against a competing surgeon's center or in favor of their surgeon, which may be false. This is why you should gather all the information you can. However, only take as fact what you have verified. You can do this by contacting INAMED or by asking for names of US bariatric surgeons and requesting of them their recommendations. You can be assured that US bariatric surgeons are familiar with the work of reputable international LAP-BAND surgeons.

Beware of Patient Herders!

Certain people are misusing the support groups and have found it easy to make a quick buck by referring patients to certain doctors. This is called *patient herding*. This is an unethical way to obtain potential lap-band patients. If you are checking out a surgeon's reputation, beware of the telltale signs of these Internet support groups. Watch for the following signs:

- Support groups that rave about a surgeon and talk bad about any other surgeon or center
- Support groups that are moderated
- Support groups that screen members before they are allowed to join
- Private emails badmouthing a certain doctor
- Soliciting on the Internet groups
- Patient coordinators that are actively searching for patients in the support groups
- Coordinators that badmouth other doctors or surgical centers
- The same group of self-proclaimed LAP-BAND experts posting to the same groups over and over
- Postings that are unfavorable to a certain group that may be deleted

As surgeons we have all had our moments in the spotlight. We have also had patients that were less than happy with us for reasons as minor as not liking the color of their hospital room. If you see support-group boards where you have never seen a single unfavorable word about a particular doctor, even something very small, it is probably one of those groups that should be avoided. There is no one surgeon or center that has completely pleased everyone in every detail. Of course, on the other hand, you should also use caution and thoroughly research a surgeon if you consistently see that there are many patients who complain about a particular doctor.

Obesity surgery is a serious lifetime commitment with our patients and in our profession and should never be taken lightly. We condemn those using support groups as a way of illicit profiteering and frightening patients. We ask those who know about this to make it public. This practice has to stop. Our feelings are shared by the majority of surgeons, the manufacturer of the LAP-BAND, and International distributors.

I would encourage all those who have a LAP-BAND as well as those investigating the LAP-BAND procedure to join one of the internet support groups listed previously in this chapter. It's a great way to meet other patients who have already had the procedure done. Many times patients will find that they live very close to each other and form small subgroups by city. Our group will also be planning future live chats with LAP-BAND experts from all over the world, plastic surgeons, and other topics that would interest LAP-BAND patients.

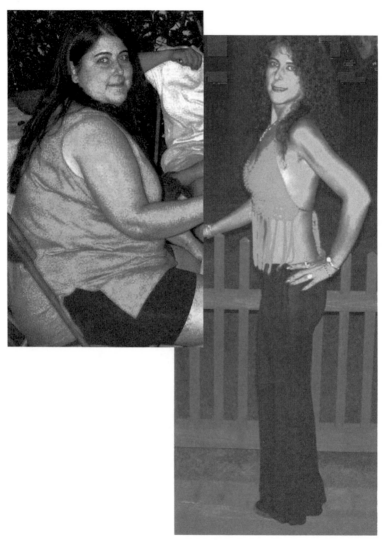

"I could hear them say, 'Why doesn't she just go on a diet?' Hey, I tried a dozen different diets. They didn't work for me. I was up to 232 and gaining. Don't let the smile fool you. I have my life back. I lost like you wouldn't believe and I feel great. I was 232 before surgery, now I'm at 125. What a difference." — Lisa Geraci-Ruppert

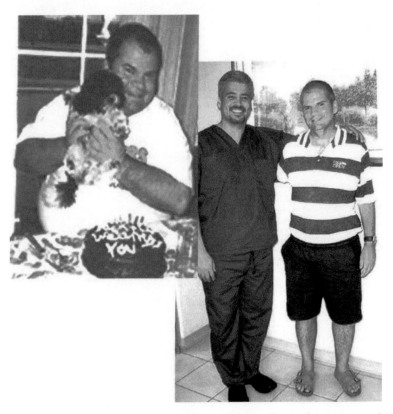

"I was fully aware that when a person is 5'9"and weighs 395 pounds,
the future is tenuous at best. I was so proud of the weight loss, I wanted
a photo taken with Dr. Ortiz and the new me." — Rick Rush

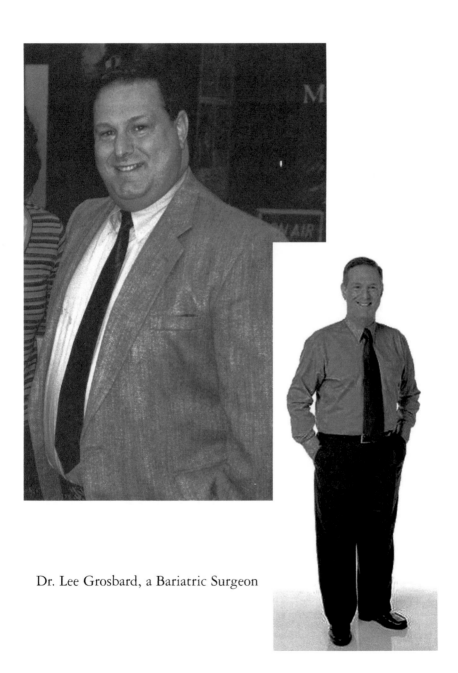

Dr. Lee Grosbard, a Bariatric Surgeon

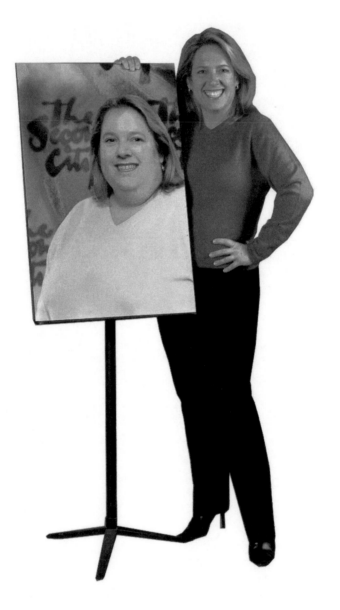

"I wanted to be invisible. People would say, 'You have such a beautiful face; if only you would lose the weight.' I tried. Then I had the band and you can see the change." — Cynthia Jones

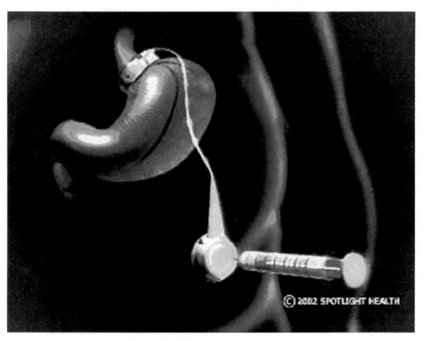

Placement of Port and Needle Fill or Unfill

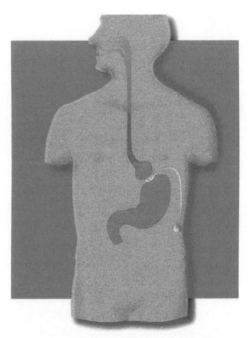

Position of the LAP-BAND at the top of the
stomach following minimally invasive surgery.

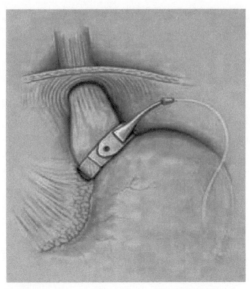

Adjustable Gastric Banding, aka, The Bioenterics
LAP-BAND® System aka LAP-BAND that has
a pouch at the top of the stomach.

6

Performing the Surgery

Contribution by Dr. Roberto Rumbaut

As discussed in a previous chapter, Dr. Belachew designed the band to be placed specifically by laparoscopy, the surgical method of making several small incisions to access the abdominal cavity with specially-designed instruments. The LAP-BAND can also be placed with an open surgery, though this is usually reserved for the extremely rare patient that does not tolerate the laparoscopic approach, or when the surgeon discovers problems inside the abdomen that require a formal incision. In any case, having an "open" surgery does not constitute a complication. It is only a change in approach and is always done thinking of the patient's safety.

Laparoscopic Procedure

With the patient lying on his or her back under general anesthesia, I approach the abdomen, either on the right side or between the legs, while other team members are positioned conveniently to assist me. The abdomen is inflated with CO_2 (carbon dioxide). We use this gas because it is nontoxic and easily dissipates from the body once the abdomen is deflated.

The inflation creates a tent-like cavity required to visualize the stomach and intestines. Imagine a tent that is collapsed on the ground; crawling in there would not reveal much of anything. Once inflated, the lifting of the abdominal tent then produces a space where it is possible to maneuver inside. Small incisions varying from 0.5 to 2 cm are created in strategic areas of the abdomen to introduce long instruments for dissection and placing of the band.

The Band Placement

Pars Flacida Technique

This is the most widely used technique in the world. This technique is named for the tunnel where the device is placed and initially accessed through a veil-like ligament named the pars flacida. It is usually safer and faster than other obsolete, rarely used techniques and results in a higher placement of the device. This technique has been related to a drastic decrease in the number of band slippages or pouch dilations that may occur.

The Stomach Tunnel

A tunnel is created just to the left of where the esophagus meets the stomach. This tunnel is created directly along the back wall of the stomach where the instrument is passed through the tunnel and where the band is pulled through. This will be its final position.

Band in Place and Closure

The band has a doughnut-like shape with a buckle and snaps back into shape once placed. This allows it to be pulled through and automatically placed into the correct position where it hugs the stomach. Due to its unique design, it slides into the buckle much like a seatbelt in a car and is adjustable for tightness. Once the band is in place, the stomach above the band becomes a small upper pouch designed to receive solid food as it is swallowed. The solid food remains in the pouch for a time, causing a sensation of fullness and prevents additional eating. Over an extended time, the solid food gradually empties into the larger stomach and is digested. As the pouch empties slowly into the lower stomach below the band, usually hours after the meal, hunger returns. Another meal is eaten and the cycle begins again.

Once the band is locked in place, several stitches are placed from upper to lower stomach. The band is sutured to the stomach wall to prevent the band from slipping. Slippage is often caused by a stomach that is redundant. How many stitches are placed is unique to each case, but usually two or three are placed there. However, certain instances occur where additional or even no stitches have been placed and still there are good results. It is a judgment call on the part of the surgeon.

Placing the Adjustment Port

Once the band has been positioned, closed, and sutured in place, the tip of the tubing is brought to the inner wall of the abdomen through one of several incisions, usually the larger incision. A pocket under the skin and fat is created to accommodate the port and is also sutured in place. A few surgeons who are considered experts in the field advocate not suturing the port. It is merely left free and sometimes results in ports that are wobbly with some flipping to the side of the wall. They handle this issue by performing all their fills under x-ray.

Even over-suturing will not guarantee that the port will stay flat without flipping, though this is a rare occurrence when it is sutured in place. If it flips, sometimes it does not need correction to return flat against the wall. At worst, a minor surgery with local anesthetic can correct this condition.

A port should be placed in an area that is comfortable for the patient and can be readily accessed by the surgeon or a medical technician. The port can be placed anywhere in the abdomen and thorax, though the most frequent location is the anterior abdominal wall. Some surgeons place the port just below the breastbone. After years of small variations, it has been my experience that the most comfortable area tends to be just above the navel midline or off to either side, but within the anterior abdominal wall.

Variations of the Procedure within the Technique

For various reasons described below, necessity sometimes requires variation from the normal procedure. Some of these techniques are so new that they are still being developed and perfected, ultimately to be shared with other surgeons for the benefit of their patients.

Tight Band and Excess Fat

Since the band only comes in three sizes, there are occasions when the band will not fit around the stomach in proper placement, for example, patients with a greater BMI, especially males with excess fat around the stomach. Precisely the best way to place the band is a challenge. Some or all of the excess fat is dissected away until the band can be closed without being too tight. The question comes up about removing all the fat; we don't remove all the fat inside the belly at the request of the patient. I get asked to do this a lot, mostly by my female patients.

Pars Flacida Perigastric Technique

Combinations of old and new, Pars Flacida and Perigastric are sometimes used. Though this sounds technical, it really isn't. Remember that we mentioned an older technique that is not used any longer or rarely? This older technique places the tunnel closer to the stomach wall but requires no fat removal. It is employed in combination with the newer technique for patients with thick, fatty stomachs to avoid immediate post-banding blockage and tightness.

Surgeons use this technique to avoid the fatty tissue that exists in the lesser curvature. Here we skip the fat that is excessive around the stomach by creating a tunnel close to the stomach wall. This results in a band that is in direct contact with the wall of the stomach that is a useful technique for the largest patients.

Hiatal Hernia Repair

When a hiatal hernia exists, it should be repaired. Once the anatomy looks normal, then the band is placed. Simply put, a hiatal hernia exists when the stomach that normally is in the abdomen slides back up into the chest. Degrees of hernias are present and are usually accompanied by a larger hiatus (the hole in the diaphragm where the esophagus passes from the chest into the abdomen).

So, the repair is simply to pull the stomach back into place and close the hiatus. During the procedure, I perform a dissecting of a hernia sac and a closing of the hiatus before placing the band. Each case is unique and the best judgment of the surgeon will determine the need for a repair. Reflux disease may co-exist, but usually is controlled once the LAP-BAND has been placed. My results coincide with others in that patients with reflux have either fewer or no symptoms after the LAP-BAND placement.

Cholecystectomy—Gall Bladder Removal

The gallbladder can be removed during the initial surgery but remains controversial. Since the LAP-BAND implant is a foreign body, it is subject to contamination, and the bile in the gallbladder can be theoretically a source of bacteria. If the removal of the gallbladder is necessary, then steps can be taken to avoid contamination. Each case is individualized.

Inguinal/Umbilical Hernia and Others Repairs

When the possibility of performing an additional surgery is evident, there is a greater risk involved, especially in higher BMI patients. Even though the LAP-BAND placement is a straightforward procedure, performing a second surgical procedure is not encouraged unless the risks are properly assessed and the need for an additional procedure is validated. Remember, all things get better with weight loss, including your health. So, if it is not absolutely necessary, we encourage waiting for a later date when weight loss has had a satisfactory impact on your health to have the second issue surgically resolved.

Previous Abdominal Surgery

Any abdominal surgery can leave scarring on the skin of your abdomen and adhesions inside the belly, creating a challenge for the surgical team and can even be an impediment to placing the LAP-BAND safely.

If a patient has had previous upper abdominal surgery, especially if the stomach was involved, then the feasibility of the LAP-BAND placement may be less. There needs to be a thorough evaluation of the type of surgery needed. Procedures like anti-reflux surgery (Nissen fundoplication) can make it nearly impossible for the LAP-BAND to be placed properly. As in any field of medicine, there are surgeons that specialize in tough cases. We have almost a decade of experience seeing and treating these cases and, though technically challenging, they can be safely and successfully done. This surgical ability, and all my colleagues will agree, comes with experience. In most cases we leave this to those who have trained in specialized fields who can determine the feasibility of difficult cases, though the above-mentioned conditions are extremely rare occurrences.

Previous Gastric Bypass Stapling

This is something new that has been reported by a handful of centers around the world, including our own. Placing the LAP-BAND around a failed weight-loss procedure is the highest technical demand and certainly not easily attempted in America due to lack of experience. There are certain risks involved. A few initial studies have reported good weight loss following a revision, though with some bands eroding into the stomach. We have performed a number of these procedures and the results are discussed in the appropriate chapter.

Different Brands of Bands

There are several different brands of adjustable gastric bands available:

- **The INAMED BioEnterics LAP-BAND®.** After extensive field trials, this is the only band approved for use in the United States. It is manufactured by INAMED Corporation of Santa Barbara, California, formerly known as BioEnterics Company. In addition to obesity products, INAMED also produces state-of-the-art breast implants and other silicone-plastic medical devices, as well as medical collagen. It has a long, excellent history and a much larger volume of bands being placed than other brands.
- **MIDBand®** is an adjustable gastric band produced by Médical Innovation Développement of Villeurbanne, France. It is considered a soft band, since it

does not have a rigid frame, as does the INAMED LAP-BAND. It is not approved in the United States.

- **The Swedish Band, AKA Obtech Band, SAGB®** is an adjustable gastric band produced by Atos Medical of Sweden under license from Obtech AG of Switzerland and currently in the FDA trials for introduction by U.S. giant Johnson & Johnson. Trials are underway in the United States.
- **The A.M.I. Soft Gastric Band®** is produced by the Austrian Agency for Medical Innovations Ltd. and is predominantly used within mainland Europe and Mexico. It is not yet approved in the United States.
- **Heliogast®.** This new band is produced by Helioscopie of Vienne, France. It has some similarities to the LAP-BAND in style. It is not approved in the United States.
- **Gastrobelt®.** This is a relatively new product from Dufour Medical in Brunoy, France. It is not approved in the United States.

Difference in Bands

- **Soft vs. Hard:** No data has proven that one implant is better than the other regarding the hardness of the material. Irregular edges and contours may be more of a deciding factor in the issue of erosions for preference of soft or hard.
- **Low vs. High Pressure:** This refers to the pressure required to fill the band and not to the pressure that the band itself exercises over the stomach.
- **Low vs. High Volume:** This merely refers to the amount of total fill volume a band can accept. Re-

striction level is reached at different volumes. Currently, there is no advantage with having a greater or lesser fill-volume band.

Size and Capacity for Each Band

The following are some figures that are frequently mentioned on chat groups and at forums: 4cc's, or cubic centimeters, 10 centimeters, 5 cubic centimeters, 9.75 centimeters, 9 milliliters.

They may be a little confusing, so let's clear up the confusion. When a number is followed by centimeters, they are referring to the length of the LAP-BAND before closing it into a ring. This varies from 9.75 cm, 10 cm, and 13 cm. When talking about milliliters (ml) or cubic centimeters (cc) they are referring to the total fill volume of a band.

Currently, INAMED released their third type of LAP-BAND in the U.S. market, the VG—short for Vanguard. This band differs from the 9.75 and 10 in length and fill volume. The previous bands have a total fill volume of 4cc, while the VG is 13cm in length and has a total fill volume of 10. It was created in response to a need for a wider-diameter band to fit those larger patients. There is limited clinical use with this new band; currently it is not intended for everybody. However, ongoing evaluations will produce valuable information. At the moment we expect no difference in weight loss or outcomes with the different size bands. Dr. Jaime Ponce of Dalton, Georgia, has the most extensive experience with the VG LAP-BAND. He has reported that the major advantage with this new model is with heavier patients. Technically speaking, it is easier to place.

For the most part, the band most often used throughout the world is the LAP-BAND that is manufactured by INAMED. At this time, it has the best track record and overall is the most effective. However, nothing in medicine is static. INAMED and other manufacturers are constantly upgrading and experimenting with new instruments for improving results.

The main purpose for having the LAP-BAND procedure is its excellent track record that gives it a decided edge in the field and allows for the best possible results when placed by a highly experienced surgical team. All surgeons are required by INAMED to go to workshops, followed by a proctorship where he or she trains under a highly experienced surgeon in this field.

Dr. Ortiz Interviews Dr. Rumbaut:

Q: Would you say the use of the Pars Flacida technique has diminished complications overall?
A: Yes, I would. They actually have diminished them drastically. For one, we see fewer pouch dilatations and, secondly, we now rarely see a posterior slip.

Q: Has this technique been widely used?
A: Just like you, I am also a consultant for INAMED, and have proctored many surgeons. Since we started teaching this technique, every surgeon in the U.S. has standardized and employed this technique, and this has obviously benefited every patient. Hopefully, complications will soon be a thing of the past.

Dr. Roberto Rumbaut Diaz is the past president of the Mexican Society for weight-loss surgeons. He is a pioneer in the field of LAP-BAND around the world and is a LAP-BAND patient himself. He has one of the busiest practices in weight-loss surgery and is director of the weight-loss surgery in the San Jose Hospital in Monterrey, Mexico.

7

After the Operation:
From the Surgery to the First Fill

(From Surgery to 8 Weeks)

From the time the surgery is completed to the time you get your first fill, it is usually about two months. Many things happen during this time. For one thing, your initial recovery takes place during those first few days. This is why we want to cover as much as possible everything you need to know and what to expect from the time your surgery is complete and when you are released to return home. There is a simple troubleshooting guide near the end of the book; it offers information that will help you get through the recovery stage.

> **Note:** The first eight weeks can determine your success or failure with the LAP-BAND. It is best to follow doctor's orders!

Recovery

Once surgery is completed and the band is in place, you will routinely spend a brief time in the recovery area. This is where you recover from anesthesia and where all bodily functions return to normal. At this point, full monitoring by the trained medical staff is essential. Keep in mind that obesity is a disease and any patient, especially the very obese, risks developing complications. Special attention is given to vital signs, cardiac monitoring, and breathing until the anesthetic wears off and the heart and lungs return to normal. In special instances, medication may be administered before or during the surgery itself to keep these and other functions in balance. When necessary, these medications are prolonged for days. This depends on any existing diseases you may have. The doctors have to be allowed time to do their work; as soon as they are ready, they will come out of the operating area to discuss with family and loved ones how the surgery progressed.

Back in Your Room

Once you are stable and awake, you will be transferred back to your room. It is here that full recovery takes place. Some patients will sleep for hours after the procedure, while others are up and about in less than thirty minutes. All patients are encouraged to sit down, then stand up, and then walk as soon as they are able. This diminishes the possibilities of lung collapse, blood-clot formation, and pulmonary embolism. The sooner you walk the better. If you are dizzy, wait until the anesthetic wears off. It's a fact that the sooner you walk, the less overall time you will spend in the hospital recovering and ultimately the better you will feel. Over half of our patients walk after the first hour, regardless of their weight, age, or gender.

Many patients ask about medications to avoid gas pain. Some patients experience two types of gas pains. There is the normal gas in your intestines that accumulates in your body after the surgery and may give you colicky pain. Everyone is familiar with these pains and gases—and I mean everyone who has ever had an embarrassing episode of releasing gas. These gas pains are frequent for various reasons. By the time you have surgery, you are required not to eat for at least12 hours. Some patients eat their last full meal (I mean FULL MEAL) the night before surgery. Often, it is referred to as their "farewell to food." It doesn't help that they usually go for the hardcore stuff such as burritos, pizza, and Chinese food. Then, too, the fact that you have a LAP-BAND also promotes intestinal gas since the band is a one-way valve that permits air to go down but not back up. All this produces discomfort after surgery. It is better known as bloating. The best treatment is to avoid it by having an empty stomach and not overeating at the beginning of the twelve-hour pre-surgical fast.

Don't, under any circumstance, eat a large meal or eat out the night before surgery; it could lead to diarrhea at the time of surgery. This is not a happy site. It is also important that you walk around as much as possible before surgery; this usually controls the bloating effect. We rarely prescribe medication to treat it. At our center, we will usually have a list of the best options, since most patients will go out anyway and dine the night before.

Note: Avoid bloating. Walk, walk, and walk as soon as you are able.

If you have a family member available or a loved one accompanying you when you take your first walk after surgery, it is helpful and safer to rely on them. If they are available, have them help you walk as soon as possible.

Those First Hours

Between the times you are fully awake until you have full mobility, discomfort or even pain may be present. This is due to having had major surgery. Even though it is a relatively painless laparoscopic procedure, over half of our patients feel mild discomfort and tenderness from it. However, there are those who feel nothing unusual. Many feel varying degrees of pain, though rarely intense. Those very few who do have intense or very noticeable pain refer to it on a scale from one to ten as a six. When the anesthetic wears off, grogginess disappears; then walking begins and pain tends to disappear.

During these first hours, you will be checked frequently by the nursing staff and doctors on call. You will be monitored for blood pressure, temperature, heart rhythm, respiration, and blood oxygen. In addition, you will be medicated with painkillers and given antibiotics to avoid infection, and also given stomach acid blockers to counteract acid secretion.

Other medications, such as blood-thinning agents, will be given to you to avoid possible blood clots and embolisms. If you are diabetic or have a heart problem, you will also be medicated as you normally are. Because of the low impact that this surgery causes to the body, most patients who have medications for any purpose are back on their usual medications the day after surgery.

As mentioned earlier, we encourage you to walk as soon as possible. At first this may be a strain, but it helps greatly to diminish the discomfort associated with your surgery.

The First Day

The exact time when the surgery is performed varies, though most surgeries are performed in the morning hours. By nighttime, you will likely have walked and sucked on ice chips or sipped a small amount of water. These are the two most important items your surgeon needs to see in order to discharge you. The fact that you have walked tells the surgeon that you have lessened the risk of complications and that you have recovered well during the first stages. Sipping water and tolerating an appropriate amount of liquid means that the band is in a correct position and is allowing liquid to pass through it. These are the two things the surgeon needs you to personally note.

High-risk patients may have to wait longer to be released because of the need to be monitored and treated in the critical care unit. Certain diseases require that the doctors treat and control these risk factors before discharging you. Two of the most common would be diabetes or high blood pressure. Others include heart problems, lung disease, and other chronic ailments.

During the first day, a patient's most frequent complaints are upper abdominal pain, tenderness, shoulder and back pain. The abdominal pain is usually compared to that of a sore abdominal muscle following exercise. Back and shoulder pain are most often caused by the gas used to inflate the abdominal area. Even though all the gas is absorbed just minutes after surgery, the irritation it causes may linger for a couple of days. This is treated by walking as soon as possible following the procedure, and taking painkillers. Back pain at times is associated with pre-existing problems such as arthritis, a degenerative disease, or a back injury. These can also be controlled by medication as needed.

Patients with a high BMI, especially men, may develop a total obstruction after surgery. This usually means the band is too tight, resulting in inability to swallow anything, perhaps even their saliva. This does not mean that your surgeon placed a band knowing that it was tight; this happens because of swelling of the lining of the stomach that takes place after surgery. All patients are prone to develop this, but usually it is the heavier males who tend to suffer the most. This is unpredictable but simple to treat. Though this obstruction is sometimes uncomfortable, there is the reassurance that it will resolve. It may take up to 72 hours to resolve, but it requires no special treatment, only patience and reassurance.

There is one positive aspect associated with postsurgical obstruction. If you experience it, you will tend to lose weight faster.

Discharge

Discharge from the center or hospital usually takes place the day following surgery. Some centers do same-day surgery, which means that after recovery, you go home. This is great for some patients, so long as they can be provided with the aftercare needed at home. We prefer to pamper our patients at least for the first day after surgery.

Patients are typically discharged from the center or hospital on the day following surgery, that is, if no complications from surgery have been noted and there is no history of co-morbidities that must be monitored during the immediate post-operative period. Your discharge orders should describe general measures, precautions, type of diet, medications, and physical activity allowed. The following is a list of requirements:

At Home Care
- Liquid diet, then solids
- Light to moderate physical activity
- Incisions cleansed with soap and water

Signs to Watch for:
- Any symptom of a complication: fever; bloating; incisions that are red, tender, have a discharge or are painful; abdominal pain; constipation; nausea or vomiting
- Any unusual physical occurrence that could signal a problem with the band

The Diet

Clear Liquids Stage

Patients should remain on clear liquids the first week. Clear liquids are water, apple juice, and beef consommé. Try these liquids at different temperatures. Some may favor warm liquids, others cold. Clear liquids are recommended because of their simplicity in the digestive process. It is important that no undue tension be placed in the pouch or the new stomach by taking anything other than clear liquids.

All Liquids Stage

You may have an additional four to seven days in which all liquids are fair game, transparent or opaque. While the dictionary may have a different definition of liquids, for the newly banded patient the definition of a liquid is whatever can be sucked through a straw. The use of a straw, conversely, is not recommended at any point of the early diet. This is due to too much air being sucked through a straw along with the liquid. You really don't want to ingest a lot of air.

Soups without meat and vegetables, such as tomato soup, are popular during this period, as are various fruit juices and vegetable blended juices, such as V8 and its generic store-brand equivalents.

Protein Stage:

The third week after surgery, the diet includes a free liquid phase that adds protein to the intake in the form of shakes or drinks. Adding protein protects your stored body's proteins. It's also a great way to kill the hunger pains associated with the phase of restricted food intake. The reason for liquids the first three weeks is to let your band heal in place.

Solid Food

This stage, hopefully, endures for the rest of your life. What should you eat to reach your weight-loss goal? Basically, you have to consume two-thirds less food. There is a good deal of information out there on proper amounts of food and types of food to lose weight. Patients need to follow the simple guidelines to sensible eating.

Food Guidelines

Here are a few *LAP-BAND for Life* guidelines that you ought to follow for success in weight loss:

- Eat three small meals a day.
- Eat solid foods (food you have to chew to swallow).
- Chew your food thoroughly and slowly from a small plate.
- Don't wash your food down with liquids.
- No liquid calories between meals.

Notice that although these guidelines mention nothing about dieting, they have passed the test of time and have been proven with the success of thousands of LAP-BAND patients. It's not expected that you drastically change what you eat just because you had the LAP-BAND procedure. You will surely eat less. What you eat may depend on your culture, customs, habits, lifestyle, and perhaps other factors. The nutritionist analyzes the types of food to eat and helps you adjust to certain types of foods to get the best results. Most surgeons offer the services of a nutritionist in conjunction with the LAP-BAND surgery. Balancing food is the key to success. Following simple guidelines and sensible selection of foods will help you reach your goal successfully.

The LAP-BAND limits the quantity of food.
You select the quality.

Note: How do I know if I am doing well? If you are following the guidelines and eating a third of your pre-surgical intake of food, you are actually doing great.

Why Liquids? Why Solids?
Why a Fill at Six to Eight Weeks?

From the time of surgery to the time of your first fill or adjustment, follow the previous liquid-to-solid diet plan, paying close attention to the guidelines by eating sensibly. If you do, you WILL lose weight. Some patients lose more, some less.

Don't worry if your band does not seem to be restrictive during these first weeks. It was not meant to be.

Your liquid phase is there to help the band heal in place. After the third week, you may go on solids, though you may want to take a little longer before trying solids. The purpose of the trial period on solids is to determine how much restriction you already have without the band having a fill.

This helps us determine the appropriate fill volume of your band. So, after the three weeks are up, you may eat solids.

During the first fill, you will usually be asked how much food you can eat compared to before LAP-BAND placement. Most will say "a lot." This means that you need an adjustment; the goal is to have you eating a third of what you would normally eat.

The band is adjusted at six to eight weeks. This is because you have had time to properly heal following surgery. During the solid phase, we can evaluate how much food passes through the band and then have an adjustment.

Dealing with Your Incisions

The LAP-BAND patient will have five incisions in his or her abdomen, ranging from about .5 to 2 cm. Some patients, especially extremely high BMI patients, will have six or even more incisions. Some surgeons use a tape to hold the incisions closed; the tape comes off after about ten days, typically in the shower. Some surgeons have moved away from using tape and apply a special type of crazy glue. A very few band patients will experience infection and/or pain in and around the incisions. The scars from the incisions are so small that, for most patients, they are virtually unnoticeable after a year. Even if scars are visible, they're not nearly as ugly as all that fat you had before surgery.

Complications

The LAP-BAND is a foreign body inside you and is subject to the reactions of your body to it. Everything in medicine involves a risk/benefit ratio. There is no clearer example of a benefit far outweighing the risks than the LAP-BAND in the fight to control obesity. With the LAP-BAND, complications are rare, usually non-life threatening, and are often resolved through laparoscopy. Furthermore, those few that do exist may be avoided by following the guidelines.

Note: Complications are avoided by following the guidelines.

Perforation of the Stomach

Though extremely rare, perforation of the stomach can occur during surgery. If it is detected during the procedure and repaired, the decision whether or not to proceed with the implant is made at that time. If the perforation has not been detected at the time of surgery, symptoms quickly arise that warrant a second surgical intervention, usually within the first 72 hours after the initial procedure. It is not possible for the stomach, perforated at the time of surgery, to lie dormant, undetected and then makes its appearance months after surgery. If perforation of the stomach is detected at a later date, it is usually due to erosion of the band or sutures.

Band Slippage

Band slippage is also known as prolapse or pouch dilatation. To understand slippage, you have to picture the LAP-BAND creating an upper pouch and a lower pouch. The upper pouch is always small unless the LAP-BAND is pushed down, creating a larger upper pouch. Much like a belt on a balloon, the lower the band is placed, the larger the upper pouch. As the band is pushed down, a greater amount of stomach is caught in the band. This may result in a total obstruction.

It is important that you understand what can cause a band slip in order to avoid this happening. Here are a few of the causes:

- **Liquid Phase Ignored.** Not following a liquid phase as indicated can put you at risk for early slippage.
- **Vomiting.** It is well known that vomiting is a common cause of slippage. This means that you avoid vomiting at all costs. Chew thoroughly, don't overeat, and never vomit on purpose. If vomiting results from stomach flu, let your treating physician know that you have a LAP-BAND so you can be treated promptly for nausea.
- **Bad Eating Habits/Chronic Vomiting.** This is well known with patients struggling with the LAP-BAND. These patients usually have a band that is too tight or simply eat too much, too fast, or do not chew long enough.

Note: Patients with bad habits are more likely to have a band slip.

As mentioned throughout the book, slippage, as with most other rare complications, is not the fault of one single event. Most surgeries are performed more or less in the same way, and when a complication arises, specific blame cannot be assigned. Typically, it is a cascade of events that lead to complications. Most of the time, a precise mechanism cannot be easily detected. Complications exist; it is a shared responsibility knowing of their existence and that they are readily treatable. You must keep your doctor informed of your recovery and evolution.

Erosion

Erosion is considered a major complication. Erosion is when the stomach is perforated by the band. This is not an instantaneous event. It is most often a slow process that takes place over time. Erosion is kind of like a worn sock. Once the heel has worn, the rest of the sock more or less stays the same. The mechanism of erosions is unknown. The only explanation is already explained: The LAP-BAND is a foreign body and as such is subject to the body's own reaction. An eroded band is a band that is being partially eliminated by the body.

We know for a fact the following:
- Erosions are very rare and tend to be fewer as experience increases.
- Erosions tend to have a benign evolution.

- Erosions are usually not an immediate surgical emergency, though they should be treated as soon as detected.
- Erosions may appear initially as an infection at the adjustment port area.
- Erosions may be totally without symptoms.
- Erosions do not seem to be associated with anti-inflammatory medications, as once thought.
- Erosions can be treated by surgical removal, repair, and replacement.

Each patient is different and responds differently to similar problems.

Since erosions do not have a precise mechanism of cause, follow the guidelines as much as possible; always consult your doctor if in doubt; and cherish your band every day of your life.

Band Infections

The LAP-BAND is a foreign body when implanted, and even though it is inert (causes minimal or no reaction), it is subject to the response of the body where it was implanted.

Bands come sterile and are placed in a sterile environment. Areas around the band can get infected, but it is unlikely that a lone, dormant bacterium is the culprit. The typical sources of contamination are two: the stomach or the skin. Once the LAP-BAND is placed, the immune system protects against infection. When there is contamination, usually it is from one of the sources mentioned. Either because an erosion occurred and bacteria from the stomach seeped out, or it is from deep in the skin pores where normal body bacteria resides. Though rare, if this happens, shifting the blame on somebody will not cure it. This is a complication inherent to all implants and should be treated properly. Patients receiving an implant should be aware of contamination.

Constant regurgitation, vomiting, and bad eating habits may also put you at higher risk for a band infection. The act of vomiting is a violent one and creates forces that could pull your stitches that hold the band in place. Not only can it cause a slippage, it may also perforate the stomach where those stitches are anchored, thus contaminating the band with the stomach liquids within. Though very rare, severe abdominal infections may develop after erosion or a pulled stitch. This often requires lap-band removal.

Treatment usually requires antibiotics and a lot of patience. Treating the underlying cause is also important. This is discussed further in the troubleshooting guide. In the worst scenario, a LAP-BAND or its port may need to be removed for a time before the infection subsides. When this happens, a few months have to pass before installing a new band.

If this happens to a patient, a repositioning of a band should not be taken lightly; all pros and cons should be discussed thoroughly with your doctor and family members present. Some opt for having another type of weight-loss surgery performed at that time.

Note: When in doubt, always rely on your surgeon. Forget about the chat groups; give yourself a fighting chance!

The Port

Detachment of the Port

Because of the forces involved inside the body, detachment of the port can happen. This does not pose a problem in itself unless the port cannot be accessed with a needle for an adjustment. Your doctor will evaluate the need to resolve this surgically. Some ports can be coaxed into place using x-ray, and since an adjustment takes a couple of minutes, the need for corrective surgery may be avoided.

Puncture of the Hose

A fill is performed either under x-ray guidance or as an office fill. When performed as an office fill, the fill is done by palpation and the needle is inserted blindly. The risk of perforating the tube that connects the port to the LAP-BAND is greater. If a puncture takes place, the band will leak. It will not hold a fill and thus become nonadjustable. A minor surgical procedure to repair the leaking tube may be required.

Tube Detaching from Port

Another very rare complication is the tubing that connects the band to the port. It can detach. Certain forces acting upon the device are involved and, though infrequent, they will require minor surgery to correct.

Leaking Band

Up to this time, no LAP-BAND has leaked because of a defect in manufacturing.

> **Note**: Most bands will leak air between the first and second fill, thus giving the impression of leaking; once all the air has been replaced by liquid, the level of fill will vary no longer.

Acid Reflux

GERD (Reflux Disease)

Acid reflux, commonly known as heartburn, is a disorder where there are stomach contents backing up into the esophagus, causing the symptom to occur. The acid burns the esophagus, causing inflammation. This, in turn, can aggravate and cause it to bleed, ulcer, or even close up. A small percentage of longstanding reflux patients will develop cancer.

Reflux (Heartburn) before having the LAP-BAND

Good news. If you have heartburn, the LAP-BAND often controls it. In many cases, the band actually cures it. So, if you have a weight problem combined with reflux disease, it is wise to have the LAP-BAND surgery procedure performed.

Reflux with the LAP-BAND

If you are experiencing heartburn after having the band, surely something is not right. Usually, it is either a band that is too tight or something has swollen the pouch and made it too tight. In any case, this is a serious symptom that should be corrected immediately. Your doctor will treat you accordingly to relieve this problem.

Over all, most patients have success with their band after surgery, that is, if they follow the guidelines to better eating, watchful care of any possible complications associated with the band, and exercise regularly. It is a marvelous tool to a better, slimmer life. So make the most of your recovery time.

Review

The first couple of months will be highly important to your success. Once you have recovered from the surgery itself, it will be important to concentrate on your diet for proper healing of the band in place. The transition of liquids to solids will come after the third week. Then concentrating on eating habits will be important. Applying the guidelines so frequently mentioned in this book will be crucial to your success. A proper fill performed at six to eight weeks will be needed to adjust the band properly and give you the restriction and fullness required. From there on, you will be on your road to success!!! And remember, the more you stick to these recommendations, the more weight you lose, the happier you will be, and last, but not least, the more your doctor will be impressed.

8

Fills—Getting the Band Adjusted
Contribution by Dr. Arturo Martinez
and Dr. Jaime Ponce

The LAP-BAND is an adjustable implant, a device with three basic components: the rigid cylindrical band made of silicone elastomer that has a built-in expandable balloon on its inner surface, the reservoir (port), and a tube that connects the port to the balloon. The balloon is inflatable with a capacity of either 4 or 10 cubic centimeters.

After a variable period, usually six weeks following surgery, the first fill or adjustment is performed. The fill begins with a saline solution injected through the port, traveling through the hose to the balloon side of the band, causing it to expand, much like you would inflate an inner tube; except that, instead of air, it fills with a liquid. When the band is inflated, it squeezes the stomach to decrease the size of the stoma or hole between the upper part of the stomach, the pouch, and the lower part of the stomach. In turn, this restricts the amount of solid food you can eat.

A key reason that there is a delay of at least six weeks before your first fill has to do with swelling caused by surgery. Surgery causes swelling of the stomach tissue. Inflating the balloon during this period could cause undue stress on the upper pouch and result in slippage of the band. For a similar reason, during the first weeks after surgery, a liquid diet is recommended. During the first few months the band has time to settle in. Over time, the swelling subsides and the tissue surrounding the stomach will form adhesions and hold the band in place.

A major concern for some is inflation of the band, intake of solid foods, and vomiting during the early period. All of these problems can be the cause of band slippage.

Does Size Matter?

Most people wear different size shoes because one size does not fit all. The same is true with the band. The INAMED LAP-BAND is currently available in three sizes: 9.75, 10, and 13 centimeters. Some surgeons prefer one over the other, but they are basically the same. The new 13 centimeter named the VG (short for Vanguard) is preferred by surgeons for higher BMI patients. At the time of surgery, if one band does not fit properly, the surgeon will remove some fatty tissue from the surgical area to accommodate the band. This can be avoided by using the new VG band.

A question frequently asked is what is the best band size? Every band is adjustable and the volume of the fill is not that significant. What is important is that it is right for you.

All bands restrict when adjusted properly, so if you have a band that fills with either 4 or 10 milliliters, don't worry. Just get it adjusted properly.

Time for a Fill

Once the six-week period has passed, the surgeon and his team will evaluate the need for an adjustment. Not all patients will need or receive an adjustment at this time. Those patients in whom the band fits snugly after surgery, usually taller individuals and/or those with higher BMIs, may take as many as eight months before a fill is indicated.

The great majority of patients require a fill at six to eight weeks after surgery.

You will have gone from clear liquids to broths and cream soups to protein that typically follows at the end of the third week when there is a transition to solid foods. Three weeks after solid foods have been introduced into your system, usually the band is ready for an adjustment to help restrict the flow of solid food.

The explanation is simple. After surgery, the simple presence of the band will cause a satiety effect, the feeling of fullness. In other words, patients are not hungry. So, the liquid phase is relatively easy to follow and the patient loses a good deal of weight, which lifts his or her spirits. By the third week, with the switch to solid foods, most of the swelling related to the surgery has subsided. At this point the band is completely deflated, but the tissue has become thinner. After the third week and before their first fill, most people find that they can basically eat anything, but shouldn't. When this occurs, there is a need for a band adjustment.

When Do You Need a Fill?

The physician needs to know if the patient is eating solid chewable foods. Since the band does not restrict liquids, mushy food such as yogurt and oatmeal slip through the stoma without restriction. This is why a wise physician counsels his LAP-BAND patient to eat only solids after the initial three-week liquid phase.

Your doctor needs to know the volume of food you are eating compared to the pre-surgery level. The goal is to restrict the amount of food that you can ingest to a fraction of pre-surgery volume. Each surgeon has a different standard as to what that fraction is. It may be as low as one-sixth to as much as one-half. I feel that one-third of pre-surgery food intake is ideal.

The second factor the physician wants to know is whether you are hungry after meals. Some patients feel hungry because they are usually eating liquids, yogurt, and cereal, and, consequently, within a few hours they are ravenous. This is a difficult habit to break. To break it, you have to eat solids. The patient who eats solid foods for breakfast will feel satiety (not hunger) and by lunchtime will not experience significant hunger to break with the recommended solid foods. In this way, the patient avoids overeating at lunchtime. Most patients who are adequately restricted will feel satiety for a few hours after a meal of solid food.

Note: Meals should consist only of solid foods, not washed down with liquids. Most LAP-BAND surgeons recommend that liquid consumption should be avoided half an hour before and an hour following the meal. Others do not prohibit drinking before a meal, and even say that drinking a cold beverage immediately before a meal will contract the stoma, which will be beneficial. Consult your LAP-BAND surgeon for his or her specific recommendation.

Before going for a fill, try to follow the guidelines as closely as possible. If you can eat more than a third of your pre-band food, you may need a fill!

Prior to performing an adjustment or a fill, the doctor needs to know if you are losing weight, how much weight, and the weight-loss pattern. The progress of weight loss is not a steady decline in regular decrements, but a mixture of sharp drops in weight mixed with periods of no weight loss called plateaus. Sheer weight loss is not the total indicator, as reduction in clothing sizes may often signal a positive trend. Remember, muscle weighs four times as much as fat by volume. The patient who has gained muscle and lost fat may be the same weight, but is losing size.

The band was designed to restrict solids, so don't schedule a fill if you have not been eating solids.

Questions to Determine
If a Banded Person Needs a Fill

Follow these guidelines and ask yourself these questions:

- **Are you eating solids?** If you answer yes, then the doctor can determine restriction level.
- **How much volume are you eating compared to before surgery?** If your answer is more than a third, you need a fill.
- **Are you hungry after a meal?** If you are hungry and you are eating solids and not washing them down with liquids, you may need a fill.
- **Are you losing weight or sizes?** If not, then you need a fill.
- **Are you exercising?** You have to exercise to protect your muscle tissue.

The Fill Procedure

Some centers offer adjustments in the office without a fluoroscope (a form of x-ray). My team and I routinely perform them using a fluoroscope; we strongly believe that an adjustment performed under fluoroscope is more objective, and that an ideal restriction level can be reached earlier with fewer visits. After assessing with questions the need for a fill, the clinician proceeds to observe the band under fluoroscope. The patient swallows liquid containing barium that tastes chalk-like, but has no effect on the stomach. As it is ingested, it clearly shows up under a fluoroscope as it passes through the band and into the rest of the stomach.

The clinician analyzes the anatomy of the esophagus: the upper pouch, the position of the band, and the tightness of the band. If the band is too loose, the clinician adjusts it by injecting the port with saline solution using a special needle that does not harm the adjustment port. A saline solution is used, as specified by the band's manufacturer, INAMED. The saline solution, which is sterile salt water, will not harm the body in the extremely rare case of leakage. Some other brands of adjustable gastric bands that have not been approved in the United States use chemical solutions that are visible on the fluoroscope. We do not use these.

How Much of a Fill Is Needed?

Every patient is different; there are different size stomachs and different amounts of fat surrounding each stomach. Just because another patient has 2.5 cc and is losing weight at that level of fill does not mean that it is the magical number that will work for another.

Some patients are steadily losing weight with no saline solution in their bands, while others have over 3 cc.

First Fill

As mentioned earlier, most patients receive a fill about six weeks after surgery. During this time, their enthusiasm is high and the surgeon and patient want to keep it that way. Most experienced LAP-BAND surgeons recommend a repurging of the LAP-BAND at the time of the first fill. Even though the band is purged of the air at the time of surgery, LAP-BAND surgeons usually find some air in the band during the first fill.

It is vital to understand why. Experienced LAP-BAND specialists have found that if there is air in the system, it will leak and part of the fill will be lost. Liquid does not leak from the band normally, but air does. Therefore, if at the first fill the band were inflated with 2 cc of saline solution and an additional 0.5 cc of air were in the system, the total of 2.5 cc will provide a good restriction. But in a couple of week's time, the air leaks out and that acceptable restriction becomes inadequate.

Note: If the original fill volume is not the same during the next visit, the patient should not panic. Usually, it means that there was air in the system. Rarely will it be a true leakage in the system that needs a repair.

How Many Fills to Get It Right?

Experienced LAP-BAND surgeons use the rule of thirds. A third of the patients will require one; a third will need two, and a third three or more. The standard protocol in the United Sates adopted by most surgeons is a gradual adding of volume. This works well, but the author prefers to get the restriction level to the correct amount as soon as possible. This can be achieved more easily with the aid of fluoroscopy.

What Does It Take to Get the Right Fill?

It is a complex process and not an exact science subject to a precise formula for fill amounts on specific days. It is more of an art, and it is one reason why experience is so important. Multiple factors are involved in the fill process, some of which have been described above. The body changes as the patient loses weight, so the fill volume that is right today may not be right after the patient has lost another ten pounds. In weight loss, everything gets thinner, including the stomach.

The right restriction is one that permits eating roughly a third of pre-surgery solid intake. (Other physicians may recommend as low as one-sixth and others as much as one-half.) A band that is too tight will not permit eating solids, and you will be forced to consume only liquids. As mentioned above, a band does not restrict liquids, so by consuming liquids and mushy foods, you will not lose weight optimally.

Fill Procedure: Non-Fluoroscope

One of the advantages of having a fill without the aid of a fluoroscope is that the fill can be performed in the physician's office. The clinician will ask a few questions before the fill to assess restriction level. The patient is usually lying down and an antiseptic is applied to the port area. The skin can be numbed with a shot of local anesthetic, though the sting of this is usually greater than the adjustment-needle prick itself. Upon palpating the port, the needle is introduced with a swift movement to access it with a special needle (Huber or non-coring needle) that preserves the life expectancy of the port. If the band is empty and this is the first fill, saline solution is injected to a certain level. No other liquid is acceptable since this is what INAMED specifies.

The protocol frequently used in the United States is 1 cc to 1.2 cc in the first fill, and then visits by the patient every two weeks where increments of .2 cc are added until the desired restriction is attained. Fills performed outside the United States are usually more aggressive.

Fill Procedure: Using Fluoroscope

This is usually performed at a radiology laboratory. Preparation is basically the same, and since the port is visible under fluoroscope, palpation is not needed. The needle is placed horizontally on the skin until the tip can be seen on the center of the port on the monitor. Once the tip is centered, the needle is stood up vertically and introduced into the port, using the fluoroscope to track progress. As mentioned above, the needle prick is slight since the needle is small.

The band is then fully inflated with around 3 cc of saline solution. If it is the first fill, to repeat, the physician or technician will purge the system of air (flushing the system with saline solution). The patient is directed to swallow special liquid containing barium that is visible under the fluoroscope, yet harmless to the body. As the barium is swallowed and travels down the esophagus, the image of it appears on the monitor. As it reaches the band, the fill technician or physician will slowly deflate the band until there is a steady flow of barium passing though the stoma. The skill is in deciding how rapid the flow should be.

Pros and Cons of Each Technique

Both types of fills are satisfactory in the sense that the patient will acquire the restriction level needed. Fluoroscopy is more expensive and requires special equipment, plus the barium that must be swallowed is not the best tasting beverage on the planet. The advantage of using fluoroscopy is that it provides an objective image for real-time evaluation, which can reveal many things about the band besides the fill level. It can show band position, the size of the esophagus and upper pouch, and, of course, the restriction level. In other words, there is a much better internal view of the band than simply a fill without visual indications. Without fluoroscopy, there may be advantages, but apart from the cost, I see no advantage of performing it without direct visualization.

The Days after the Fill

Once the fill has been performed, the band will be tighter. You will not feel it, of course. The urge to eat the same amounts at the same velocity will be there, but the ability to do so will not. Typically, due to inattention, you may ingest food that has not been chewed well enough. When this occurs, you will often experience PBing, or Productive Burping. This is not a burp, but a regurgitation of food that backs up into the mouth from the lower esophagus. In the worst case, repeated PBing may erode the inner lining of the esophagus, and you will not be able to eat solids for an indefinite amount of time. However, in time, you will revert back to normal food intake.

In the most serious reactions to the PBing effect, the treatment is an emergency deflation of the band, along with a ten-day liquid diet and acid blockers to help the swelling go down. It is for this reason that when the patient has a fill, many LAP-BAND doctors recommend consuming only liquids for three days.

What Indicates the Need to See the Doctor?

- **Not losing weight early on, even though you are eating solids.** At around six to eight weeks, most people will not have any restriction and can eat anything. If so, they need a fill.
- **Feeling no restriction just after a fill.** The patient has had a fill, felt restriction at first, but then suddenly no more restricted feeling. What happened? The band can readjust in its position slightly; the fill volume can also change slightly (not considered a leak; it is just a tolerable permeability of the band); or the body also thins out, either totally or just at the area where the band is located. The patient should not blame self or the doctor; it simply means that there is a need for another follow up fill. How soon? Usually in a couple of weeks, though some bands do tighten up with the mechanisms discussed earlier. This is why a couple of weeks' wait is good.
- **Chronic vomiting.** If the patient wants to eat solids and every time the patient tries to eat solids, it comes back up, this is due to either a tighter fill than needed or something has triggered a swelling of the stomach wall. This can only be resolved by deflation of the band. If the restriction is too tight, the band will damage the stomach lining further, and the patient will be forced to go on a liquid diet, during which time the

patient will not lose weight. More importantly, this can trigger a major complication, such as slippage.

- **Plateau.** The patient should analyze if he or she is losing sizes, though the weight does not drop. In this case, the patient should wait awhile; it is just a redistribution of fat and muscle tissues. A little exercise will help. It will actually kick start the metabolism.

Checklist If You Are Not Losing Weight:
- Are you eating solids three meals a day?
- Are you chewing thoroughly, not feeling full, and eating around a third of the volume of your pre-band intake?
- Are you selecting your food judiciously?
- Are you not losing weight or sizes?

If the answer to all of these is yes, then you need an adjustment!

---

*Not **wanting** to eat solids is the patient's choice; not **being able** to eat solids is a different matter that requires medical attention.*

Scenarios: When a Fill May Not Be Needed

Not Eating Solids

Eating solids means losing weight. If you don't want to eat solids, the LAP-BAND will not help you loss weight. This is a decision that you must make. Consuming liquids will not produce weight loss. It is strongly recommended that a patient who is not eating solids be in contact with the surgeon and staff for counseling to solve this problem, which may be a symptom of a more serious underlying issue.

Reflux Symptoms

Reflux symptoms are caused by inflammation of the stomach lining and usually occur after you have recently had an adjustment, or there has been an episode of food dislodging, PBing, and vomiting. Treatment for this is a self-imposed liquid diet. Unfortunately, after the banded person has reverted back from the liquid diet and returns to eating solids, most will fall victim to the same bad eating habits that caused the swelling. They ultimately will need band deflation. Otherwise, at the fill level of the band, eating solids will continue to irritate the stomach. If the physician does not deflate it, the banded person is condemned to a liquid diet in which he or she will not lose weight. So deflation is the safest way to go.

To give the mucosa a rest, the doctor may prescribe an acid blocker and liquid diet for anywhere from five to seven days. By this time, the stomach lining should be back to normal. Soon thereafter, a careful readjustment of the band is initiated. Often, counseling and habit modification are of utmost importance to achieve weight-loss success.

Band Tightens and Loosens During the Day

Typically, the band is tighter in the morning. Acid contact during the night can cause temporal thickening of the lining and, thus, greater restriction. Two or three glasses of water before breakfast can help smooth the way for solids. Keep away from extremes such as very hot or very cold foods that can trigger esophageal spasm and further prevent you from eating an adequate breakfast.

Some banded people cannot eat for a number of hours after rising, no matter if they drink hot liquids or not. They generally compensate by having breakfast at lunchtime, lunch at suppertime, and supper in the late evening. There is no right schedule with the band.

The fill is a vital part of band management and you need to be aware of the correct tightness at all times. Also, the fill is an essential part of the overall success of the weight-loss journey and needs attention by your doctor to reach the goal you want to achieve.

Review

If I could tell you something that will guarantee your success, it would be to follow the guidelines.

We eat to enjoy food and feel full, plus the other small detail about nourishment. So, eat until you are full. The band will prevent you from over-eating if you eat solid foods. Enjoy it. It sounds simple and it really is.

Dr. Ortiz Interviews Dr. Martinez:

Q: How important is the adjustment after the band for weight loss?
A: It may be the most important weight-loss factor. Feeling the restriction and being able to eat less and still feel full is what helps patients lose weight. Other factors are less important.

Q: Most patients want a very tight fill. What is your opinion on this?
A: I think there is a very thin line between being correctly adjusted and too tight. If patients are eating solid food and cannot tolerate even a third of their former intake, they are definitely too tight.

Q: Are there any risks involved in having the band too tight?
A: Yes, absolutely. We have seen slips develop after a band that was too tight and not loosened promptly. If a patient's band is too tight, they switch to a liquid diet and, in turn, not lose weight. So being too tight is actually bad for the patient.

Dr. Ortiz Interviews Dr. Jaime Ponce:

Q: You prefer performing the fills under x-ray. Why is this?
A: We find that we are more efficient. We have an average of three fills per patient in the first year. Without fluoroscopy, our average was as high as ten fills in the first year.

Q: Do you see patients reaching restriction sooner when performed under fluoroscopy?

A: Yes, most feel restriction after the first fill. We use this technique because we find ourselves performing fewer fills, but they are more effective.

9

Guidelines and Nutrition
for Success
Contribution by Dr. Gabriela Miranda

I have always said it is easier to walk a straight line than swerving all over the road. You will still reach your goal, but one is much faster and shorter in the long run. The same goes with the LAP-BAND. You can try it the surgeon's way or not. Many patients try it their way at first. Sooner or later, they will end up following the guidelines that have passed the test of time. We start out with the now modified *Ten Rules for Success*, originally developed by Dr. Paul O'Brien of Melbourne, Australia and Dr. Rudolf Weiner of Frankfurt, Germany—two of the leading LAP-BAND surgeons in the world and personal friends.

1. Eat only three small meals a day.
2. Eat solid foods, slowly, and chew thoroughly (approximately 15 to 20 times a bite).
3. Stop eating as soon as you feel full.
4. Do not wash down your solids with liquids.
5. Do not eat between meals.
6. Eat only good quality foods.
7. Avoid fibrous food.
8. Drink enough fluids during the day.
9. Drink only low-calorie liquids.
10. Exercise at least thirty minutes a day.

Let's examine each of these rules and understand why they are important:

✓ **Eat *only* three small meals a day.** Once the LAP-BAND is properly adjusted, you will require only small amounts of food to reach fullness. By eating three meals a day, you will fill your pouch, feel full, then allow enough time to empty it to feel hungry again, and then you repeat the cycle. You only need to fill the pouch three times a day with appropriate food to give the body adequate nutrition.

The size of the meals will be dependent on the type of food you eat. The LAP-BAND is designed to restrict solids, not liquids. So the combination of eating solids and an adequate fill volume will determine the size of your meal.

✓ **Eat solid foods, slowly, and chew thoroughly.** Many patients have a difficult time with solids during the morning hours. If this is the case for you, open up your band by starting with a couple of glasses of liquids before your first meal. Eat solid foods slowly and chew thoroughly. The band was designed to restrict solids. A normal meal for anybody is typically composed of mainly solids. This means we want you to enjoy what you eat. A properly adjusted band will permit you to eat only a third of the volume of food you were used to eating.

The brain takes 20 minutes to detect that your stomach is full. Since your new stomach is now your upper pouch, this smaller space is filled by less food. Eating slowly will permit you to fill it to an acceptable level without overdoing it. It will also permit you to enjoy your food thoroughly with less quantity, more quality.

Chewing thoroughly will permit you to eat adequate amounts of food. If you gobble and neglect to chew your food thoroughly, pieces of food will not go through the stoma and will clog the pouch. (Think of a pebble clogging the hole in an hourglass, preventing the sand from falling.) You will soon learn that chewing thoroughly is very important. When an excessively large piece of food clogs the stoma, then your body reacts in a way that feels quite unpleasant. It will create a good deal of viscous saliva (many call this thick solution "Slime"). You will feel like you ate a baseball, and you may become slightly nauseous. The nauseous feeling and pain will increase, and most banded people find they have to vomit, but not the violent vomit common before surgery. It will be a pinkish goo that is regurgitated.

This condition is popularly referred by LAP-BAND patients as "PBing" or "Productive Burping," though this is not a burp. Following one of these episodes, it will be a while before you feel like eating again.

✓ **Stop eating as soon as you feel full.** Because you are eating slowly, you can detect when your pouch tells you that it is full. Stop. Push the plate away. Just because you CAN shove more food in, doesn't mean you should. Stuffing is a hard habit to break. Remember, your band can be at risk if you push it to its limit.

✓ **Do not wash your solids down with liquids.** The reason being, liquid creates a slurry of food and allows it to slip down the stoma faster, which defeats the goal of getting the pouch full in order for the hunger signals to turn off. We have heard for years the phrase "wash it down" as in "wash those cookies down with milk." It is wise not to drink within twenty minutes before a meal, and an hour after. Some recommend taking 2 hours after a meal before drinking. Many surgeons think it is acceptable to drink right up until a meal starts. Some banded people, eating out, drink ice water or iced tea until the food comes, which may have a beneficial effect of tightening the stoma.

✓ **Do not eat between meals.** If you have been eating three regular small meals of solid foods and are properly adjusted, you should not be feeling physical hunger. You may have psychological hunger, also called head hunger and emotional hunger, but it is not real hunger. See Chapter 10 to examine possible causes of psychological hunger and ways to defeat it.

✓ **Eat only quality foods**. There is a wide variety of good quality choices for your daily regimen of food intake.

✓

It surprises me how people are sometimes scared to eat six slices of whole wheat bread or six tortillas a day, but do not feel a bit guilty eating five tablespoons of ranch dressing over their salad, (lots of calories, lots of fat). That is a bad choice. It is simple, check the food in a food pyramid. Here are some samples of preferred food and foods to avoid:

Cereals:
- Prefer grains like beans, lentils or whole wheat bread, or oats.
- Avoid pastries, fried rice, cakes and pies.

Vegetables:
- Prefer broccoli, brussel sprouts, cabbage, carrots, cauliflower, corn, cucumbers, eggplants, leafy greens (spinach, collard greens), mushrooms, onions, peppers, pumpkin, tomatoes, and winter squash.
- Avoid french fries, tempura vegetables, potato salad.
- Prefer fresh fruit, one piece for breakfast, one at lunch, and one for dinner. Try apples, apricots, blueberries, cantaloupe, grapefruit, kiwi, oranges, plums, pears, watermelon, and mango.
- Avoid canned fruit, dried fruit, and coconut.

Meat, poultry and fish: A serving is the size of a deck of cards; most people need two to three servings a day. 1 Serving = 2-3 oz; a day = 5-7 oz
- Prefer light meat, poultry, fish, shellfish, legumes, egg whites
- Avoid hotdogs, bacon, peanut butter, sausage, duck, fried poultry

Milk, cheese and yogurt: Two servings a day, three if you are a teenager or pregnant or a lactating woman.
- Prefer nonfat and 1% milk, low fat cottage cheese, nonfat yogurt.
- Avoid whole milk, whole cheese, whole yogurt, milk shakes, and ice cream.

Fat: You do need fat. Three servings a day is good.
- Prefer avocado, vegetable oil, almonds, and nuts.
- Avoid mayonnaise, lard, butter and margarine.

✓ **Avoid fibrous food.** Certain vegetables (asparagus) and fruits (pineapple) and some meats contain many fibers that may clog the LAP-BAND, even if they are thoroughly chewed. Eating these can only cause regurgitation and vomiting. This, in turn, can upset the normal function of your band.

✓ **Drink enough fluids during the day.** You should drink at least six to eight glasses of fluids per day. Many banded people drink a great deal more. As the body burns off fat, it creates waste products that must be eliminated. The fluid intake is critical to providing a channel for excretion of these waste products through the urine. Again, drinking should be done at least twenty minutes before and an hour after the three daily meals.

✓ **Drink only low-calorie liquids.** Drinking water, tea and coffee without milk and sugar, and other non-caloric beverages, are acceptable. Many banded people have found Crystal Light to be a satisfying alternative. Consuming carbonated beverages are for the most part not encouraged.

✓ **Exercise at least thirty minutes a day**. This rule is very important. Physical exercise consumes energy and sustained exercise increases your metabolism. You can start off slowly with walking and using a pedometer walk 10,000 steps a day and then gradually add more strenuous exercises, such as joining a dance class, yoga, or whatever is of interest to you that will offer you vigorous exercise.

Nutrition and the LAP-BAND

Once your LAP-BAND is in place, you will be on a liquid diet for three weeks. This requires you to be a compliant patient and have no solids during this phase because, if you eat solids, your pouch will likely enlarge, or if you start eating too soon after your surgery, you may experience regurgitation (Pbing). Or even worse, you may cause your LAP-BAND to slip out of place.

On your fourth week with your LAP-BAND, you will start with solid food, and it is important for you to have three solid meals a day. Learn to sit down at a meal; take your time and enjoy every bite. Remember to chew thoroughly. Always try to use the best quality food available.

Go back to the basic food pyramid; all the foods you need are there. Try to erase from your mind those magic diets that work only for a period of time and then when you go off, you regain the weight and more. THERE IS NO MAGIC! Just good quality food choices. That's it, and it is all found in your food pyramid.

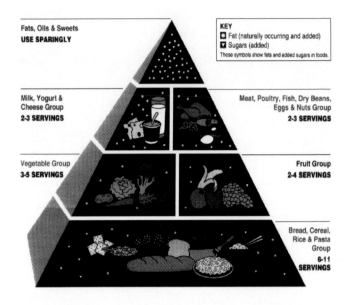

Carbohydrates

The base of the pyramid is composed of carbs. Your diet should have 50-55% of your total calories in carbohydrates. This means that a considerable amount of your energy should come from the carbohydrates you are consuming. Carbohydrates provide energy for the brain and are stored in your body in a special way that can be used for energy purposes. However, even though carbohydrates are the energy source for your body, if your diet exceeds the amount of carbohydrates it can store, it will then turn into fat. There are two kinds of carbohydrates: complex and simple.

- Complex Carbohydrates: These are the carbs you should prefer in your diet, you can find these carbs in good healthy foods such as cereals, whole grain oats, vegetables, legumes, and some fruits. These are foods rich in vitamins and fiber.

- Simple carbohydrates: These carbohydrates are sugars that are found in fruits, honey, corn syrup and other sources of sweets. Milk also contains carbohydrates in the form of lactose.

One gram of carbohydrates equals 4 calories. Here is a breakdown of carbs in the bread group.

One serving of the bread group equals:

- 1 slice bread
- 1 corn tortilla
- 4 crackers
- ½ cup cooked rice (half size tennis ball)
- ½ cup cooked pasta (half size tennis ball)
- ½ cup cooked beans
- ½ cup cooked oatmeal
- ¾ cup cereal
- 1 baked potato (that fits in the palm of your hand)
- 3 cups popcorn

Protein

Proteins are made from amino acids, also known as the building blocks for protein. There are two kinds of protein: the one in the diet and the other in the body.

Foods that contain protein are poultry, eggs, meat, soy, fish, nuts, beans, and vegetables. Protein can provide energy only to certain extent. When a person fails to eat enough carbohydrates and lacks enough carbohydrates stored in the body to be used, at some point the protein has to take over the job of carbohydrates and supply the energy the body needs. This robs the body of muscle.

The purpose of proteins is for building and repairing tissues. You can find protein in your nails, hair, muscle tissue, bones, and red blood cells. Proteins also facilitate chemical reactions.

The body needs protein in the amount of 15-20 percent of your total dietary intake. This is not usually the way most people provide for their bodies. A lot of people eat a great deal of protein, more than the body needs. Check what part of the food pyramid the chicken, beef, and eggs occupy. It is on one of the middle levels, not the base.

One gram of protein is equal to 4 calories. If a person eats more protein than needed, it will not store in the form of larger muscles. However, some chemical reactions may happen and it will be stored in the form of fat.

For an average adult, it all adds up to 3 or 4 servings of the meat group a day. It is really not that much.

One serving from the meat group equals:
- 2-3 ounces cooked lean meat
- 2-3 ounces cooked fish
- 2-3 ounces cooked lean poultry
- 1 slice of turkey ham
- 1 egg
- 2 tablespoons peanut butter

Fat

Body fat is stored due to excessive calories. It could be from carbohydrates, proteins or dietary fat. A healthy body needs dietary fat to make tissue and manufacture hormones. Body fat protects the organs and gives shape to the body (breasts, hips). Dietary fat should be no more than 30% of your total daily calories.

One tablespoon of fat provides 120 calories. One gram of fat provides 9 calories. No more than 10% of your total daily calories should come from saturated fat.

Saturated fat may damage your arteries. You will find these fats in butter, coconut, coconut oil, red meat, and whole milk dairy products. This unhealthy fat may contribute to raising your low density cholesterol level (LDL), and an excess consumption of saturated fat can also raise your triglycerides.

- Transaturated fat: This is made from non-saturated fat and has been through a chemical process called hydrogenation, where oil is turned into a fat-like margarine. They act very much like saturated fat. Another word used for transfatty acids is "partially hydrogenated vegetables;" be alert when you are reading food labels.
- Monosaturated fat: This helps reduce bad cholesterol and raises healthy cholesterol in the blood. Some examples are canola and olive oils, and avocados, peanut butter, walnuts, and almonds. Even so, use them in small amounts, because they are fattening.
- Polyunsaturated fats: These lower blood cholesterol and prevent heart disease; some of these food choices are corn oil, soybean oils, and fish oils.

One serving of fat equals:
- 1 teaspoon oil
- 1 teaspoon margarine
- 1 teaspoon mayonnaise
- 1 teaspoon butter
- 1/5 avocado
- 2 tablespoons nuts and seeds
- 1 slice bacon
- 1 teaspoon regular salad dressing

Beverages

During the first months after surgery, try to avoid carbonated drinks; these drinks could cause your band to slip. In addition, avoid high-calorie drinks, like frapuccinos and milkshakes. These drinks will pass perfectly well through the LAP-BAND, but they won't help you drop the weight you are trying to lose. Instead, drink low-calorie drinks, and use artificial sweeteners for your coffee, or your fresh lemonade, or sugar free fruit juices.

Remember that alcoholic drinks are rich in calories, so I suggest no more than one drink a day. Try to keep well hydrated because if you are dehydrated, the body won't be in the optimal condition to lose fat.

Let's take a patient for an example. Forty-four-year-old Edna had her LAP-BAND placed and lost 30 pounds with 50 pounds more to go to reach her weight goal. But she stopped losing the weight even though she had a LAP-BAND fill and was eating very small amounts of solids. She spoke to the nutritionist and realized that she was consuming too many calories via liquids. She was having juices, and whole milk and even some ice cream. Of course, when she stopped bypassing the LAP-BAND, she lost 9 pounds the following week.

You should eat from all of the food groups every day. I recommend to my patients a very practical tip that I refer to as *The Plate*.

The Plate

Divide your plate into four sections, leaving the center for the following results.

- In the first box put a serving of protein, poultry, fish or red meat (the size of your palm or the size of a deck of cards).
- Put your green veggies in the second box (you can eat as much as you want; eat at least ½ cup)
- In the third box, there should be some fruit (remember fruit and veggies prevent cancer).
- The fourth box should contain one or two servings of carbohydrates, or one or two starchy vegetables (corn, carrot, potato, or yams). I recommend you eat your carbs at the end of your meal, because some people have trouble eating carbs with the LAP-BAND. In this way, if you have difficulty eating with the carbs, you've already eaten protein, fruit, and veggies.
- In the center of your plate should be one serving of fat. Remember that monounsaturated fat is best.

Use cooking spray instead of oils or margarine for preparing your meals, or cook in the oven or grill or boil your foods. Don't deep fat-fry your meals.

You need to have two servings of dairy products daily, but since these are liquids, eat a non-fat yogurt as a snack between breakfast and lunch, and have a glass of skim milk or a cup of non-fat frozen yogurt between lunch and dinner.

Eat from every food group at each meal. This will provide your body with more of a variety of nutrients. You should try a little bit of every choice even though you can't finish what is on your plate.

If you feel like eating something more between meals, try something fresh like a fruit or vegetables. Avoid snacking on foods from a bag (chips, chocolates, cookies). Try cucumber, a fruit, or salad.

WHAT COUNTS AS A SERVING?
Food Groups

1 slice of bread	1 ounce of ready to-eat cereal	1/2 cup of cooked cereal, rice, or pasta
1 cup of raw leafy vegetables	1/2 cup of other vegetables, cooked or chopped raw	3/4 cup of vegetable juice
1 medium apple, banana, orange	1/2 cup of chopped, cooked, or canned fruit	3/4 cup of fruit juice
1 cup of milk or yogurt	1-1/2 ounces of natural cheese	2 ounces of process cheese
2-3 ounces of cooked lean meat, poultry, or fish	1/2 cup of cooked dry beans or 1 egg counts as 1 ounce of lean meat. 2 tablespoons of peanut butter or 1/3 cup of nuts count as 1 ounce of meat.	

What passes; what does not pass

It is well known that people differ from one another with what are known as problem foods due to the LAP-BAND. This is normal. Some people have problems with breads and some with red meat. This isn't the end of the world if you do have a problem with either of these. All you have to do is substitute what you can't eat for something in the same food group.

Let's take Jacob as an example. He has a LAP-BAND and he doesn't tolerate bagels or bread. He went to the nutritionist and found out that potatoes can be part of his regular diet, and also that potatoes are a good source of carbohydrates. Jacob took a potato and chopped it, and then cooked it with some cooking spray on the grill. He got his non-fat french fries that were easy to swallow and still a good source of carbohydrates. He also was glad he was allowed to have some crackers.

You need to be wise in your selection of food. Always try and obtain the finest foods on the market and be cautious in your preparation so as to bring out the flavor without excess calories. If you truly follow the guidelines presented here, you will lose weight.

10

Hunger, Pains in My Brains?
(One patient's point of view)
Contribution by Sandy Johnston (LAP-BAND Patient)

Anyone who has gone as far as having a consultation visit with a bariatric surgeon or attending a weight-loss surgery seminar has heard the statement "weight-loss surgery is just a tool and you must do your part." This is true with the LAP-BAND as well. While the band curbs physical hunger, it does not address all of the reasons we eat. The band does, however, give us time to think about what we are going to put in our mouths before we do it and also allows us the time to realize that we're full. What I mean by this is that the band takes away that insatiable hunger that tells us, "I must immediately stuff something in my mouth or I'll die!" This allows us to think about what we are going to eat and ask ourselves, "Do I really want or need to eat that?" The band doesn't allow us to mindlessly stuff ourselves at such a fast pace that we don't even realize that we "ate the whole thing" without knowing it!

Does the band always stop us from putting something we shouldn't in our mouths? Does it always make us stop eating when we're comfortably full? Will grazing be a thing of the past? Will the band make us hate the taste of chocolate and ice cream? Unfortunately, the answer to all of these questions is no.

Let's talk about the psychological reasons we eat. This is what we banded people call "head hunger." Let me give you an example of head hunger that I experienced and that I'm sure anyone who has battled a weight problem will relate to.

My mother makes the best cakes in the world. Our friends and family members always ask her to make the cake when it's someone's birthday. Of course, she made the cake for my son's birthday, her famous 4-layer chocolate and vanilla cake with buttercream frosting. I was too busy at the party to have any. But, later that night, when no one was looking (because we all know that if no ones sees it, it doesn't count!), I served myself up a generous slice of cake complete with a scoop of ice cream.

I decided beforehand that no matter how long it took, I was going to eat that cake! I started to eat. The pain hit at about the fifth bite. I knew I was too full to continue to eat that cake. I was furious! I decided that I would just wait a little while and have a sip of water to wash it down faster. I took another bite and then came what I call, *cake revised*. Yes, no one was watching, no one except my band! My band has eyes and ears! Did my stupidity end there? Of course not!

After I threw up the cake, I tried to eat more! Luckily by then, the cake was not as appealing as it was when I started.

The heavier we become, it seems the more we depend on food. Everyone has their own psychological reasons for eating, but for most, the reasons are many. Food is comfort, food is a companion, food is something to do, food is celebration, and food is enjoyment. Food can help dry your tears, help you forget that someone made you mad, help you deal with a stressful situation, and the list goes on. Food is your best friend; food is your worst enemy. Those reasons don't magically end when you get your band, but the band does allow you to separate physical from head hunger.

Now we have a band, now what? What are we going to do when someone makes us mad? We have two choices: we can still find something to eat that will easily go through the band, like ice cream maybe, or we can learn another way to deal with the situation. (Okay, maybe we have three choices. We could hit that person with a gallon of ice cream!) We won't always make the right choice, and that part is still a struggle, but at least with the band we can learn to deal with one thing at a time. We can work on focusing on our solving our head hunger issues and not have to worry about physical hunger.

It's amazing, when I really pay attention, how little physical hunger I have now. I used to hear thin people say really stupid things like, "I was so busy today I forgot to eat!" I used to wonder how anyone could *forget* to eat! Now I know. Keeping busy is probably one of the best ways to lose weight with the LAP-BAND. It's better and more effective than worrying about how much protein you ate today or how many calories were in your lunch!

Sometimes when we choose to eat when we're not hungry, it's just out of habit. You don't automatically change something that you've done for maybe all of your life just because a doctor put a band in your body. We still need to stop and think about why we're going to put something in our mouth. Some find that writing down their feelings at the time they want to eat or keeping a diary of what they're eating is helpful. Even doing this for a few weeks or days can be a real eye-opener. We all have to find what works best for each of us.

It's also helpful to plan ahead and have a few activities on hand that you can do, like sewing, painting or any kind of hobby that requires you to work with your hands. Try leaving reminder notes of things you've been meaning to do on the refrigerator for those times when you find yourself standing in front of it ready to attack its contents. Many times it's just a matter of engaging in something to distract you for a short time to realize that you're not physically hungry. Someone also suggested hanging naked pictures of yourself, front and back, (OH MY!) on the refrigerator door as a deterrent.

Frequently, we have to deal with social eating. There will always be holidays, weddings, and parties where food is there and someone will want you to eat it. Will you appear rude if you don't eat the type or amount of food that someone else thinks you should be eating? Maybe. But do you really care?

This brings me to the next issue we have to contend with: the opinions of our loving family and friends. There will be those who have very strong opinions of weight-loss surgery in general. Most of them don't mind sharing those opinions with you, whether you want them or not. This is where you have to be strong! You don't *owe* anyone an explanation of why you feel the need to consider or why you had the surgery. You can choose to *offer* an explanation, but that is your choice.

I chose to tell all of my family, friends, and acquaintances about my surgery. I simply told them that this was something I needed to do to save my life and live a quality life. I have a disease for which I wish to seek treatment. Maybe this treatment is not for everyone, but it's for me! I have not always received positive reactions, and in fact, my choice was even used against me on one occasion in an attempt to make me look like an inadequate person. I have also come to realize that I can't change the fact that ignorant people exist out there.

Did I change or did everyone else change? Those of us who have struggled with the disease of obesity don't usually stop to think about what the psychological effects of weight loss will be. We're so busy looking for the answer that we don't have time to think about what's going to happen after the weight starts coming off. And frankly, we don't care. We just want it gone! During my pre-operative visit with a nutritionist, she said something to me that I, at the time, discarded as ridiculous. She said, "You will lose a lot of friends because of this surgery." I thought to myself, "Come on lady, you don't know what you're talking about! I am a middle-aged woman with middle-aged friends." I thought that this kind of behavior would only apply to teenagers, not people my age! *My* friends and family would be happy for me and they would all support me. After all, I couldn't even walk un-assisted anymore, I couldn't breathe and walk at the same time and I couldn't even participate in normal daily activities. Why in the world anyone would NOT support me in this? Guess what? She *did* know what she was talking about.

If you take a closer look around, you will see all different kinds of people in your family and circle of friends. You'll see people ready and willing to help and support you throughout your weight-loss journey, people that are jealous, people that are just waiting to try to sabotage your weight loss, and maybe even a husband or wife that would feel more comfortable and less threatened if you remain fat. You'll see former eating buddies that will miss you, people that don't believe you can do this, people that don't want you to do this because you might be successful, and other people will ask them why they haven't done it, and people that are mad because you're not the invisible fat woman that they used to push around. You now have a spine! Some people won't like your newly found spine.

There are many times in the lives of obese people when we've accepted and even become accustomed to inferior treatment by others. We work extra hard at the office in an attempt to prove that we're not lazy, and never refuse to do someone a favor, in order to be liked. Even as kids, we let other kids copy from our paper at school in order to be liked or accepted. Of course we always tried to be first to make a fat joke before someone else did. We have to be funnier, work harder, be smarter, be more helpful, and generally do whatever it takes to feel better about ourselves, even if it includes letting others take advantage of us.

All this changes when you lose weight. You will first start to notice it with people who didn't know you before you lost the weight. Maybe it's something small like someone striking up a conversation with you in line at the grocery store or asking you for directions. You're not invisible anymore. Do others see you differently, or do you see yourself differently and present a different, more approachable image? There are different opinions about this subject, but one thing is certain, whatever happens, in addition to feeling better and being healthier, your life will change.

Some of us will find the courage to leave a relationship and some will rekindle one. Some people acquire enough self-esteem to find a better job or ask for a raise. Most of us discover that we are worthy people with talents, feelings and souls just like everyone else and we don't have to accept the inferior treatment that we once did in order to be accepted or tolerated by others, especially those who were disgusted by us. But most of all, we begin to notice the other fat people who are still suffering. We want to run up to them, throw our arms around them, and tell them that we know their pain and there is a way out of that pain. But we also know that we can't do that. They will have to find their own way in their own time.

What is the difference between men and women and obesity? Obesity does not know gender, but it is said that 80% of people that undergo weight-loss surgeries are women. Why? Women still associate their looks with their self-esteem more than men. I'm not saying that men do not suffer from self-esteem problems due to their weight, but let's face it, men are visual creatures and when they're in a room full of people, they will notice a woman's looks long before they have been introduced. Women are also very critical of other women. We are sometimes our own worst enemy. I have heard women say very mean things about other women. This doesn't seem to be as common for men. Still, men are start-ing to seek the answer to treat their own obesity. Men tend to do very well with the LAP-BAND and almost always lose weight much faster than women.

Review

In summary, while the LAP-BAND is not the magic wand that the surgeon waves in front of you and makes you thin, it is currently the closest thing we have right now. Some days are still a struggle with the dreaded "head hunger." Almost everyday is still a struggle to get out there and exercise, but the complete loss of the physical hunger forever is truly a dream come true for an obese person.

I'm someone that started with a very high BMI and my weight-loss journey will take longer than the journey of others with less weight to lose. I haven't finished my journey yet, but I will get there. Not a day goes by that I'm not thank-ful for my LAP-BAND, for my surgeon, and happy I had this surgery. I'm also thankful that I found out, by accident by the way, about the LAP-BAND. Unfortunately, many people in my shoes end up with a gastric by-pass without even knowing that the LAP-BAND exists. They will have to run the risk of problems from malabsorbtion, bowel leaks, and other terri-ble, life-threatening complications. Some people have asked me when I will have the band taken out. My answer? "NEVER!"

11

Insurance Reimbursement and the LAP-BAND
Chapter by Velma Moreno-Bandy

One of the major challenges with having the BioEnterics® LAP-BAND System® performed in the United States is getting insurance coverage for the procedure. Several major insurance companies have denied coverage for the LAP-BAND, claiming it is still experimental/investigational. However, those same insurance companies pay for the more expensive and invasive Gastric Bypass procedure while not recognizing the differences between open and laparoscopic approaches. After making the difficult decision to have obesity surgery, many would-be patients come to realize that they have to perform additional tasks to get their insurance carrier to cover the LAP-BAND.

It is interesting that health insurance carriers claim the LAP-BAND is an experimental procedure when the LAP-BAND has been performed in countries around the world for more than 10 years. Also interesting is that many countries have banned or refused to do the Gastric Bypass surgery that has the historical backing of surgeons in the United States. These surgeons still refer to the Gastric Bypass surgery as the Gold Standard. With an increased death rate from complications with the Gastric Bypass surgery, this standard "should" be reviewed. From a strictly economic standpoint, you would think insurance companies would welcome the LAP-BAND for its increased safety and documented track record of controlling obesity.

There are those who feel insurers are worried that once they provide coverage for the LAP-BAND, hordes of obese persons will clamor for the surgery because of its increased safety, relatively short recovery time, and long-term health benefits. Insurers may be betting that those who need weight-loss surgery are too frightened of the outcome of the more invasive procedures to attempt approval. Yet in reality, it would benefit the insurance companies to have their increasing numbers of plan members opt for the LAP-BAND surgery and avoid the costly results of associated lifetime illnesses that are so prevalent with obesity.

Several of the more progressive insurers are gradually beginning to cover the LAP-BAND. However, members with some plans must meet very stringent qualification criteria (such as excessive waiting periods of as much as three years) that can cause many members to simply give up seeking insurance approval.

Steps to Take in Obtaining Insurance Approval

You may speed up the insurance approval process by contacting your insurance company by phone or via the internet to determine if the LAP-BAND is a covered procedure. Even if they say yes, you may discover that obesity surgery is covered only if you meet certain weight, age, or health-related illness conditions.

And you may also find out the insurance company is not familiar with the LAP-BAND procedure. They may be confused and think you are referring to Gastric Bypass surgery. You must be specific in what you say and how you ask your questions. It is sometimes helpful to call back a second time to verify that the information you received is accurate and request documentation.

If you do have an insurance benefit for obesity surgery, it is often up to the patient to advise the surgeon of the information required for the insurance approval. By going to a qualified bariatric surgeon, chances are the surgeon and his office staff will assist with this process, but they often do not have the time or resources to take full responsibility of negotiating with your carrier.

Insurance companies frequently request relevant medical records that document any co-morbid conditions or diseases with a plan member's obesity. The following is a list of weight-related co-morbidities, which simply means other illnesses besides obesity that are impinging on your health. These that are listed are in no special order of importance to your health:

- Diabetes
- Osteoarthritis
- Sleep apnea / obesity hypoventilation syndrome
- Cardiovascular disease
- Hypertension
- Lower extremity venous stasis disease
- Dyslipidemia
- Urinary stress incontinence
- Gastro-esophageal reflux
- Idiopathic intracranial hypertension
- Infertility

Many insurance companies also require you to have participated in a medically-supervised weight-loss program, which usually includes weight-loss medications. By law, your medical records belong to you, so you have every right to request and receive them in a timely fashion. You should request your medical records from all doctors you have seen within the past 5 years, whether or not you think they will help you obtain insurance approval for your surgery.

Your medical records should consist of chart notes, lab reports, doctor's letters, previous prescriptions, etc. Whether you've seen an internist, cardiologist, pulmonary specialist, psychologist/ psychiatrist, orthopedic surgeon, or other specialists, make sure you request copies of all your records. Even with all these records, it may take a few weeks or longer before your insurance company makes a decision on whether to provide insurance coverage for the LAP-BAND surgery.

Patients should collect all available records from their commercial weight-loss efforts such as Weight Watchers®,

Jenny Craig®, and Diet Center® etc. In some cases, these records may be difficult to get if the center has closed, moved, or appears unavailable. All records from physicians for medically-supervised programs are important to gather, as these records provide your weight at most visits, what medications you were given, dietary regiments, etc.

It can also benefit you to have a current list of clinical literature, articles, news releases, and such to demonstrate to your doctor that you have done your homework. This information may also support the efforts of your surgeon when submitting your pre-authorization paperwork.

Pre-authorization Materials

To expedite receiving a pre-authorization from your insurance carrier, it is imperative that you've done your homework in contacting your insurance and collecting the specific criteria that you will need to meet as part of their review. This information will be important to your surgeon and his billing team.

You should work closely with your surgeon's office in providing them with all the necessary information and supporting documentation referenced above that they will need in order to prepare a letter of pre-authorization for submission to your insurance provider. Remember, your surgeon's office may not have the resources in place to do all the leg work for your individual case.

Every insurance company that covers the LAP-BAND procedure has specific criteria that need to be met when requesting approval. Some may require a psychological evaluation as part of the initial review—get it done! Some may require a dietary evaluation—get it done! By not providing the specific criteria, you only delay the surgical approval and/or receive a denial, therefore, requiring you to initiate the tedious process of appealing. It is important to **always** provide the necessary information the first time around!

Below is a list of the basic information and support records that should be included in the pre-authorization letter:

- Height and weight
- Body Mass Index (BMI)
- Specifically identify all of your co-morbidities (related illnesses)
- Chart notes and records from all doctors you have seen for previous attempts at weight-loss in the last five years

When submitting your letter of pre-authorization, make sure it is sent by whatever service is available to your surgeon's office (Certified Letter, Registered Mail, Overnight Delivery) that provides a tracking source. This expense may be your responsibility, but provides your only proof of delivery.

Support Groups

Patients should participate in local or internet support groups before surgery. These patients have already experienced similar insurance issues and may be able to provide you with information that specifically pertains to your insurance company. You may get information on the criteria you need to qualify for the surgery. This could include the name of a primary care physician who is an advocate and supports obesity surgery more than your current primary care physician. Maybe it is the name of someone with your insurance company who is supportive and can assist you in expediting your approval. Whatever they can provide is helpful; they are your allies.

Documenting

Patients should share responsibility and work closely with their surgeon's office, following their guidelines in making periodic calls to the insurance company on the status of your predetermination letter. Do not call the insurance company every day, as you will only annoy them. Calling once a week is reasonable since processing your pre-determination request can take approximately 10 to 30 days, sometimes longer. Be patient, yet diligent.

Both patients and surgeon's need to be aware that verbal requests for coverage are not valid and that a request must be in writing. You have to submit your request in **writing**! Any conversations you have or information you acquire verbally from your insurance carrier needs to be DOCUMENTED. Make sure you get the first and last name of the insurance person you are talking to. In most cases, your surgeon's office will usually keep an insurance tracking log in your patient chart of all communications with your insurance carrier during the approval process. This is always good practice.

Available Sources of Information

One of the best sources to gather information on the LAP-BAND is the internet. You can find numerous websites, chat groups, email support lists, etc. Just remember that there can be misleading and incorrect information out on the web, so don't be afraid to question and confirm what you hear. Your best source of information will always be from your personal consultation with the surgeon. Make sure to take a notepad and a list of questions you may have. Take advantage of the resources available to you in learning all you can about the benefits and risks of any surgery, as well as the possible after effects from other patients.

Locating a Surgeon for the LAP-BAND

To locate a surgeon who has been properly trained and credentialed by INAMED, the manufacturer of the LAP-BAND, we recommend that you go to their web sites at www.lapband.com or www.INAMED.com. You will be able to locate surgeons, by state, who are qualified to perform the procedure. You then have the ability of consulting with as many of these surgeons as you feel necessary before making a decision on which surgeon to choose. Do your research.

Appeals and Grievances

If you receive a denial for surgery from your insurance provider, all is not lost. Don't simply stop because of an exclusion clause. Fight for your right to have coverage. Review your medical insurance policy as well as the letter of denial carefully. Each insurance policy provides a certain number of appeal levels. If you feel they should provide coverage for the LAP-BAND surgery, then fight for it.

The following are helpful tips when fighting your case:

- Make a list of your questions when interacting with your insurance company. Make sure you are specific in your questions.
- Make sure your policy clearly defines the appeal levels and process. If not, contact them directly and continue to ask questions until you receive all the information you need. Ask them to send it to you in writing.
- Make regular calls to your insurance provider, and write down with whom you spoke.
- If you don't receive a return call, send a fax explaining that you wish to have someone speak to you about coverage for LAP-BAND surgery. Continue to phone and/or fax until you receive a return phone call.
- Don't give up. You have every right to appeal your denial.

What Other Options Do I Have?

The following are options to consider:

1) Ask your surgeon to submit your appeal through the INAMED Hotline run by *Weight For Life®* www.weightforlife.com. The INAMED Hotline is a **free** service to all surgeons who have been trained on the LAP-BAND for assisting them in acquiring pre-authorization for the LAP-BAND as well as appealing denials. *Weight For Life* ® has over 12 years of extensive experience in working with insurance companies nation-wide in acquiring pre-authorization and fighting appeals.

2) If an individual patient should choose to contact *Weight For Life®* for assistance, they can access them through www.weightforlife.com to discuss available services and fees.

3) Contact your local or regional support groups. Members may have already gone through the struggle for coverage and won. Consult with them. They will usually be glad to help you navigate through the bureaucratic path toward getting approval.

4) With limited number of appeals, you may want to consider hiring an attorney experienced in dealing with obesity-related insurance denials and/or grievances.

How do I find an Insurance that will cover the LAP-BAND Surgery?

It is difficult to answer this question since insurance companies do not broadcast that they provide specific coverage for obesity surgery and unless you change your job, you would need to find an individual plan which would require a great deal of research on your part.

When Insurance Coverage is Not Obtainable

When insurers simply will not cover your LAP-BAND surgery, you may want to look at other ways to finance your surgery. LAP-BAND surgery can run between $15,000 to $30,000 in the United States, and less in Europe and Mexico. You should check with your surgeon to see if he or she offers financing services, possibly consider obtaining a personal loan through your bank, taking equity from your home, searching the internet for healthcare financing companies, or other financial sources. If an international program is selected, make sure it is an approved LAP-BAND System with designated follow-up support.

Success Is Possible

Regardless of your present circumstances, it is possible to secure help with your fight for coverage. It may take time, preparation, and patience on your part in dealing with your insurance company.

You have to be persistent if you want to win!

12

LAP-BAND over Bypass
in Rescuing a Failed Weight-loss Procedure
Contribution by Dr. Rudolph Weiner

Failure to lose weight or regaining weight after Gastric Bypass and other stomach stapling is a frequent problem. Again, Europe, Australia, and Mexico are pioneers in performing LAP-BAND surgery to rescue failed bariatric procedures, namely, the Gastric Bypass and other stomach stapling. The application for the LAP-BAND is approved in the United States for clinical use.

Why Stomach Stapling Fails?

Though an easy answer would be just to blame the patient, nothing could be further from the truth. We are faced with a number of factors. First of all, when somebody has weight-loss surgery, they have it mainly because they have tried other non-surgical weight-loss methods without success. Once you have the surgery, the intention is to limit either the food quantity or the absorption of it, thereby losing weight. Though this may seem fail proof, it is not. Something that is highly difficult to calculate and counteract is the marvelous ability of the body to adapt. Because of this adaptation, the body can change drastically as it is met with challenges.

Picture this scenario. You have a patient that has had a procedure that restricts. When surgery is performed and the technique is followed to perfection and a patient has lost all of his or her excess weight in the first year, and then slowly regains most of it by the third year, then something went wrong. What? Perhaps body adaptation from the simple change in eating habits, to the avoidance of "dumping" caused by sweets, to the ability of the stomach to expand as time goes by to accept more food, combined with the ability of the esophagus to push the food down with greater force and challenge any restriction. Even the intestine, which is not designed to be a stomach-type sack, slowly enlarges and accommodates more and more food. Microscopic changes in the intestine also happen, adapting to the changing needs, absorbing nutrients where no absorption normally took place. How in the world can you blame the patient for this?

I am personally a true enemy of calling the patient a failure. Yes, maybe you have regained all the weight, but if anything, I would call it the body's success over weight-loss surgery!

For an adapting patient, we need an adjusting procedure!

Why the LAP-BAND Works

The LAP-BAND provides a physical limit to the amount you can eat. When used to rescue a failed weight-loss procedure, it acts exactly like it would on any first-time recipient.

By placing the LAP-BAND in the highest part of the stomach, the first thing the food will meet, after passing through the esophagus, will be the band. Any stapling previously performed will usually be left below the LAP-BAND placement. Patients having the LAP-BAND after stomach stapling will rely on the LAP-BAND for restriction and not their previous stapling. Any other residual function of the previous surgery will be left intact. Patients having dumping with sweets because of an original Gastric Bypass will be left exactly with the same effect once the band is in place. Only restriction will be added.

Am I a Candidate?

A failed procedure usually takes place after the first couple of years have passed since the original surgery. The obvious manifestation is weight gain. Most patients also experience an increasing ability to eat with little or no restriction whatsoever.

Candidates are patients that have had previous gastric stapling (Gastric Bypass, vertical banded gastroplasty, etc.) and have gained most of their weight back.

To be a candidate, a patient should also be able to eat a lot. If a patient still has restriction from the previous surgery, the band will not offer more.

Preparation

Though every single pre-surgical step is similar to a first-time LAP-BAND recipient, there are certain tests that have to be performed in order to accept the patient for surgery.

The most important test is the Barium Swallow. This test provides an image under x-ray of the anatomy of the esophagus and stomach. We want to see what type of surgery was originally performed and how it has changed over time. This gives us a general idea of the feasibility of the procedure.

Other tests are also important, and we decide upon additional tests or evaluations once the general status of the patient is assessed. Don't get me wrong. This might look simple in writing, but the actual surgery is a complex process due to the following:

- Obesity and coexisting disease
- Unusual anatomy due to previous surgery
- Extensive abdominal scarring
- Disseminated intrabdominal adhesions

This is why selection of the candidate and preparing that patient for surgery are steps that can increase the chances for success.

The Technique

The technique involves certain steps that are not considered during a typical LAP-BAND placement. For one, we have extensive abdominal scarring when the original procedure was performed by an open approach. This means our laparoscopic incisions' positions will vary from the usual placement. Another challenge is the intra-abdominal adhesions. It requires time and skill to take down these adhesions to expose the surgical field where the band is to be placed. Once we do expose this area, we find tissue that has scarring and is harder to work with, and again, requiring extra care for successful placement of the band. As the dissection proceeds, the visualization of the structures and anatomy become evident. This also permits a final analysis to decide if the LAP-BAND can be placed at that time or not. So, usually, it will take us a couple of hours of surgery before we can actually determine if the patient will end up with a LAP-BAND or not.

The reasons for this are due to the possibility at any time during the surgery of finding circumstances that would prohibit us from positioning the band. Some patients may not have an adequate anatomy. Some others have so many adhesions that proceeding with the placement would be a greater risk. There is also the possibility of contamination from the intestines into the abdominal cavity. This is because extensive scarring can adhere firmly to the intestines, and the risk of inadvertent perforation is much higher.

Every test needed to determine if the LAP-BAND placement is feasible is performed before surgery. It is only at the time of surgery that this can be definitely decided.

Results

To date, we have performed over thirty LAP-BAND placements over a previously failed surgery. All surgeries were performed through the laparoscopic approach without the need of a formal incision. All surgeries were completed with no complications and had the LAP-BAND successfully placed. Most of our patients are six months to two years out of their

LAP-BAND placement. Weight loss has been comparative to the other bariatric patients, with weight loss surpassing 50% of the excess weight lost.

Though to date we have had no major complications detected, recent publications report a higher incidence of erosions into the stomach. Dr. Rudolph Weiner from Germany has reported a 7% incidence of erosion. We have yet to see this, but we caution every patient of the possibility of this happening.

Review

The LAP-BAND placement over previous weight-loss surgery is a recent option for patients with a failed procedure. It has been performed around the world successfully, but higher erosion rates have been reported. In our experience, this procedure may be successful by adhering to strict selection criteria: a work-up, and the surgical procedure. As long as the benefits outweigh the risks, this procedure has something to offer. The higher incidence of erosion has to be addressed and studied so we can avoid it.

Dr. Ortiz Interviews Dr. Rudolph Weiner:

Q: Professor Weiner, where do you see the major advantage of the LAP-BAND over other weight-loss procedures?
A: The primary advantage of the LAGB (Laparoscopic Adjustable Gastric Banding) is an extremely low risk of postoperative leaks, bleeding, and wound complications, including infection and hernia.

Q: How about the super obese? Do you consider the LAP-BAND as a feasible option?

A: The lower excess weight loss of LAGB in contrast to the combined procedures led to a tailored concept in bariatric surgery, which indicates for super obese LRYGB (Laparoscopic Gastric Bypass) or LBPD-DS (Laparoscopic Biliopancreatic Diversion with Duodenal Switch) as a single-step treatment. Otherwise, our results in super obese patients have shown that LAGB is feasible and successful in patients with higher BMI.

164 LAP-BAND For Life

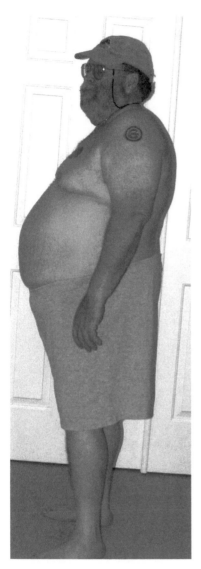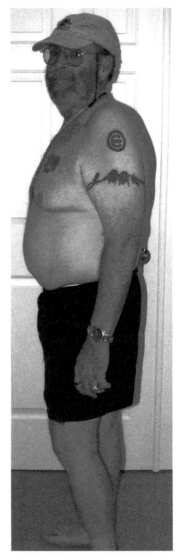

"The lowest I ever got on any diet was 240, then up again to over 300. I wore pants with a size 58 waist and a 4X shirt. I was kidding myself, thinking I could do it on sheer willpower and the latest diet. Losing it was finally possible with the help of my lap band. I now weigh in at 240 and I'm still losing. At 61 dressed up, I look much like other men in a room of mature men." — Dan Lester

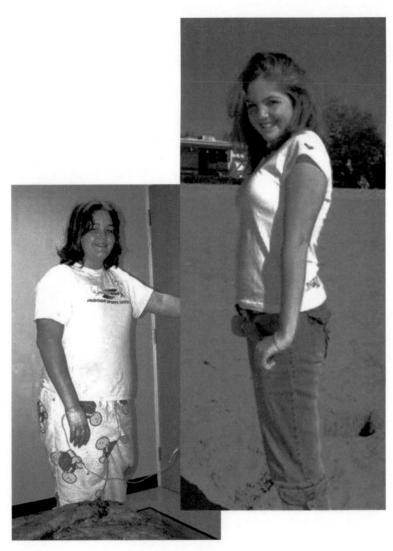

Cassie Divello at age 13

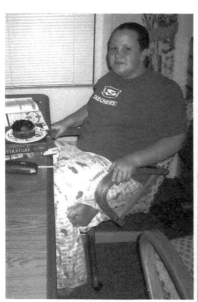
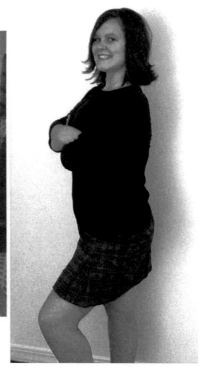

"I hit rock bottom! I was so depressed and just ate nonstop out of emotional stress. I was only 13 and weighed 228 pounds. I lost 50 pounds after surgery. Doing it at this point in my life made perfect sense, and I have absolutely no regrets about having had the surgery!" — Shanae Scott

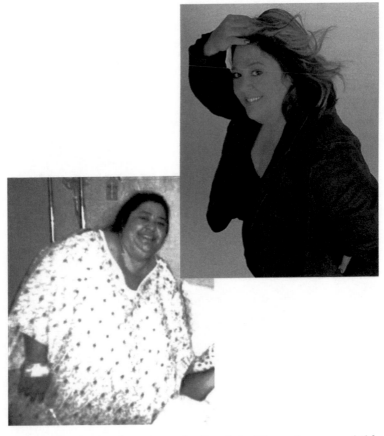

"I was a fat child, a fat teen, and a fat adult. Throughout my child-hood was teased and taunted. Since my surgery, I've gone to Disneyland without a wheelchair and I've gone camping with my family. I'm not afraid to go places that will require me to walk a distance."
— Sandy Johnston

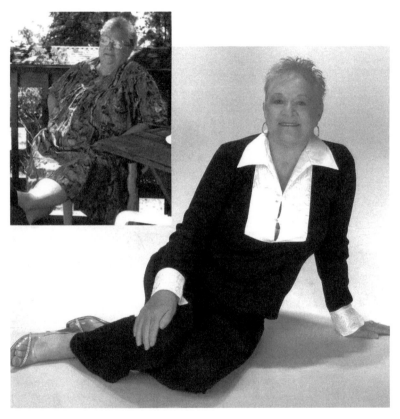

"It wasn't easy getting around. Let's just say I was grossly overweight before my saving surgery. Two years later I posed for this photo of the new me. Friends say I look 15 years younger. I feel 20 years younger after my lap band." — Gayle Muller

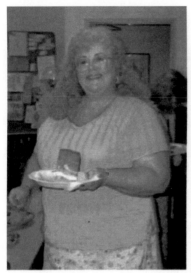

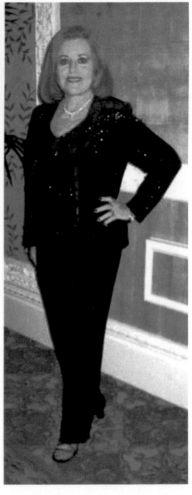

"I loved food and was always hungry and it showed. Something had to happen to break the trend where I was topping out at 255 and hating it. After my safe lap band surgery by Dr. Ortiz, I have dropped to 152 and will shed even more to reach my goal of 130." — Carolyn Williamson

13

LAP-BAND for Adolescents

The LAP-BAND has a promising future with special patients. Now that more than a decade of experience has passed and after perfecting the technique, this procedure has been proven to be safe and effective. This opens new possibilities in its application for weight loss in various arenas. One of the most desirable aspects is that it is gentle and mild enough for adolescents. After surgery, they are so resilient and vibrant that they recover rapidly.

We live in a society where one of the most affected obesity age groups is that of the adolescents, with numbers growing dramatically out of control. Measures have been taken at every level to stop this rampant disease. Fifteen percent of American children age 12 to 19 are either overweight or obese, according to the 1999–2000 National Health and Nutrition Examination Survey, up from 11% a decade earlier and 5% in the late 1970s.

LAP-BAND for Adolescents

This is a very special program that is starting to develop in select centers around the United States. The LAP-BAND has not yet been FDA approved for clinical use in this age group. Experience in adolescents started originally in Australia, Europe, and Mexico. Dr. Fielding in Australia has placed the LAP-BAND on over fifty teenage patients with good results. I have also performed the LAP-BAND on two dozen teenagers ranging from 13 to 17 years of age in the last three years with good results. I'd like to explain my findings and pass along information based on this handful of teenage patients in these select centers around the world.

The Candidate

An obese young person is difficult to define because of active growth. Adult parameters are still valid for adolescents. The excessive accumulation of fat defines obesity and is what causes the appearance of early diseases such as diabetes, hypertension, and other diseases normally seen in middle-aged people. Teenagers with a BMI of 35 to 40, with a comorbidity, are the ones needing the LAP-BAND. Some specialists are advocates of a stricter requirement—50 BMI—for young people to qualify as candidates for surgery.

This is not a static issue. Take note that these indications in teens are rapidly evolving and currently being redefined. This is the research and evaluation not only of surgeons, but pediatric surgeons, endocrinologists, and other specialists as well. They are taking part in this change of attitude toward help for youth. Pioneering work in obese adolescents is ongoing at NYU Medical Center with the help of Dr. Christine Ren, Bariatric Surgery Program Director, and Dr. George Fielding, who has vast experience in this field, both of whom are sure to set the standards in years to come.

The Preparation

Though it may sound aggressive, drastic problems require drastic measures. In the case of obese adolescents, we don't support the use of the Gastric Bypass for weight loss, since the LAP-BAND has proven to be safer and just as effective. When I refer to the adolescent as a candidate for surgery, I'm not speaking of kids who are simply chubby, but rather those who are outright obese. Most of my young patients have a fully developed skeletal structure at 13 to 15. Typically, those in this age bracket are young girls who reach maturity at an early age. Boys, as a rule, reach maturity at 16 and 17. Apart from being physically mature, mentally they understand their weight problem and want to resolve it.

During the workup, my patients are seen by a pediatrician, psychologist, and nutritionist and assessed by other specialists, if needed, prior to surgery. These specialists determine if surgery is warranted and treat any co-existing disease, if needed. It is surprising to listen to obese teenagers who have simple and straightforward requests such as, "I'm fat. Please help me lose weight!"

Not only does the teenager require multiple evaluations, it is equally important to involve the parents in the decision. I have performed the LAP-BAND on teenagers whose parents have had a weight-loss procedure and understand the benefits. With most parents, it was Gastric Bypass surgery. It's interesting, however, that all requested the LAP-BAND for their child. This was, in part, due to the safety of the procedure as well as the reversibility, should the child someday opt to have the band removed, which I'm convinced is not likely to happen if the young person going into adulthood has learned how to deal successfully with the band.

The Procedure

The surgical approach is not a great deal different with an adolescent than with an older patient. Most of our young patients have a fully-developed body and, therefore, the technique described in the appropriate chapter for adults is applicable to the youth. It is vital that the teenager understands exactly how the procedure is performed and what to expect after the surgery. Special attention is given to the teen's early mobilization and adherence to the liquid diet.

The Results

Recovery for youngsters is much the same as with adults, with the exception of intervention by a pediatric specialist who will be involved with follow-up exams and medical examinations. Adjustments are performed at six to eight weeks following surgery, and follow-up visits will determine the need for further adjustments. I have not seen any difference in weight-loss progress with youth as compared to adults. Adherence to the guidelines is similar, with one very important added benefit, that of concerned parents who work closely with their child, with the surgeon, and with the pediatric specialist. All work as a team to make the procedure a success. It's amazing to watch concerned parents and know that they are a stabilizing influence on their teenager.

Web Support

Because of the need for LAP-BAND surgery at an early age, groups of adolescents on the Internet support sites are growing in numbers. Those who had the band mention that they are on their way to or have reached their target weight loss. You can sense the enthusiasm of these young people and observe how suddenly they want to share their newfound place in their teenage social circle. Young people receive encouragement and tips from LAP-BAND centers set up specifically to assist young people in achieving their goals.

Support for these patients is crucial and is given by the team of experts handling these patients at each center. A wonderful source for support and information is on the Internet in the form of moderated support groups for adolescents, helping these youngsters exchange their experiences, difficulties, and challenges on their way to success. Go to the following site to see what I mean: www.lapbandforum.com.

Review

My staff and I are carefully selecting, preparing, and performing surgery on these young patients with great success and follow up. We've done follow-ups where we have recorded results and have made them known to other young people who inquire. So far, like other groups, we have had very promising results in this age group that desperately needed or need the LAP-BAND. You need only read how Shanae and Cassie feel about their experience to sense the importance of an obese young person who has lost excess weight.

Shanae Scott Thrilled with Her LAP-BAND Surgery

"My name is Shanae Scott and I had the LAP-BAND Surgery at the age of thirteen. I was a normal weight infant but became chubby as I got older, and I was already obese by the third grade. Watching (or hearing about) everything I ate became my way of life.

By my teen years I had been on many fad diets and convinced my parents to let me try "*just one more*" infomercial® miracle weight-loss or exercise program, but when my grandpa, whom I loved deeply and was extremely close to, passed away, I hit **ROCK BOTTOM!** I was so depressed and just ate nonstop out of emotion. I got on the scales one day and had reached 228 pounds, and that made me sink into a deeper depression. The reality of it all hit me hard, but I was simply out of control.

My mother knew where I was heading with my weight because she had a Gastric Bypass surgery twelve years earlier. My mom lost a lot of weight with her bypass surgery, but has gained much of her weight back. She will suffer the rest of her life now with health issues she has because of having that Gastric Bypass surgery. She was adamant that I would never, ever have surgery for weight-loss, but once I became so depressed, my parents were desperate to find a way to help me. My mom did some research on obesity and found out all the new things they were working on and learned about the LAP-BAND surgery. Because of the differences in the LAP-BAND and the Gastric Bypass (mainly, the fact that if there was a problem, they could just take it out!), my parents decided it would be safe and said that I could do it (along with a little *pleading*, of course!).

We looked into getting the surgery done in our home state, but nobody would even consider it until I was 18. I can only imagine how much heavier I would have been in five years at the rate I was gaining. My parents were really nervous about me having surgery in Mexico, but Dr. Ortiz was willing to meet with us, and after we met with him, he felt I was mature enough to handle the surgery, and my parents felt it was safe.

I had my LAP-BAND surgery six months ago and I have lost fifty pounds with fifty pounds to go. I realize I still need to watch what I eat and how important exercise is to reaching my goal weight. Yeah, it's hard to go to a sleepover when everyone is pigging out on pizzas and sodas, but I am feeling better about myself all the time, and that is better than the taste of the best pizza! I now have **HOPE.** The LAP-BAND surgery has made it possible for me to finally get my weight under control.

Although I have not reached my goal weight, I actually have a chance at a normal adolescence. I am a freshman now and I'm feeling more confident all the time. I am kind of a shy person anyway, and being so heavy kept me from making new friends. I would never even have considered talking to a guy. I'm gaining the confidence I need to change all of that. I'm getting compliments all the time on how much better I look. Also, I'm grateful to my parents for supporting me in having this surgery, and that Dr. Ortiz did it. I'm trying out for Dance Company next year, and I'm looking forward to school dances and activities. Being a teenager is hard enough, but being an obese teen is an *excruciating heartache*!!

I have never believed in being obsessed with worry over a few extra pounds. I really think it is silly for people to have unnecessary surgery because of a few extra pounds when they try to be *perfect*, but I think it's fair to want to be *normal*. I want to be a normal, with a healthy weight. I want to get married and have children and live a healthy adulthood.

Because of all the positive traits of the LAP-BAND surgery, I can have it adjusted to assure my weight-loss will continue. I can have it adjusted when I choose to give birth, or I always have the option to simply remove it if there is ever a problem. Doing it at this point in my life made perfect sense, and I have *absolutely no regrets* about having the surgery! The scars are no big deal, and I have had no complications at all! The LAP-BAND surgery simply gave me a chance at a happy adolescence and a healthy adult life."

— Shanae Scott

Cassie's Excitement with the Results of Her LAP-BAND

"My name is Cassie, and I had my surgery March 17, 2004. I was only 13 years old. At surgery I weighed 218 pounds, and now I am 155 at 5'7".

First I want to say, 'I AM SO HAPPY.'

My life seemed to be on hold because of my weight. I did all kinds of sports and the weight still kept coming on. I tried dieting and went to the nutritionist and it still didn't help. I was gaining weight very fast every month. I became more and more depressed with every unsuccessful diet.

My mom did some research and found Dr. Ortiz and Dr. Martinez at the Obesity Control Center. She explained everything to me and let the final decision be up to me. I was scared but, at the same time, ready and wanted my life to change, and to be like the other kids and enjoy sports once again and the cute clothes. I had my surgery and the very same day, I was up, out of bed, and walking. The next day, I left for home. I am back into sports and many school activities, not to mention my grades are great and I have lots of fun friends. If any teen would like to talk me about the surgery or just needs support, I would be happy to chat with you by email. Thanks for my life back."

— Cassie Divello

Don't be misled into thinking that only those over eighteen can have the surgery. When kids in their teens are 100 pounds overweight, the social and physical problems can be enormous. They have a right to become svelte like so many of their peers. Don't settle for less than you can have. Get the weight off and start living.

Personal Note

This is a very personal note from the author. When I performed surgery on Shanae, I had a long chat with her and her parents. It was so refreshing to meet her and to listen to why she was considering the LAP-BAND. Simply put, she said, "I want to live a normal life and be thin." And, of course, we told her we could help her in reaching her goal.

When I read her contribution to this book and saw these pictures, it brought tears to my eyes. I have never felt so fulfilled or proud of a patient as I do with Shanae; she is an example to follow, for both young and old. She is my greatest achievement. Thank you, Shanae, for helping inspire others in reaching their goal. Thank you for inspiring me even further to do what we do.

14

Life after the LAP-BAND

The ultimate goal for every LAP-BAND patient is that, after a year and a half to two years, they have pretty much reached their ideal weight. At this point, their eating volume should be a third of what they were used to before the band and, hopefully, they have acquired a feeling of fullness on a small amount of food. At this time, usually patients have reached a new baseline that permits them to enjoy less food and keep the weight off. What then? Well, typically most patients vary little from their new weight level, though with greater effort, they continue to drop the weight. So, what is involved in a LAP-BAND maintenance diet once patients have reached their goal? Let's take a look.

Reaching Goal Weight

Actually, the latter part of this book explains this very concept of reaching the weight goal. Currently, we have a combination of medical knowledge, experience and common sense. Just a note here: a condensed version is also available by reading those chapters that deal with the formula for success that comprises two simple rules:

1. Follow guidelines (to the letter)
2. Get adjusted (see your doctor when needed)

I'll explain in greater detail what is meant by these two essential rules that, if you strictly adhere to, you will drop the pounds.

Following Guidelines

People are as diverse as life itself. Unfortunately there is no perfect formula for each person undergoing LAP-BAND surgery, and I seriously doubt that any medical doctor has one. We have also learned that most people trying to lose weight detest dieting, hate restrictions, and are sick of rules. So, if you have an idea that patients getting the LAP-BAND are very unlikely to follow a strict regimen, you are probably correct. By the same token, we have also learned that a strict diet after the LAP-BAND is not essential to reaching a weight-loss goal. A solution to this is to offer the patient a few guidelines to adhere to, something akin to a LAP-BAND to create limits, meaning food intake and adjustment. If you follow these guidelines and fine-tune the band, it will work and you'll arrive at your weight-loss goal. Sounds simple? It is just that clear for many patients. This is how most banded patients reach their goal.

Getting Adjusted

Having a fill will not work if you fail to follow guidelines. The band only restricts solids that are eaten three times a day. Mushy or liquid food will pass through the band and add calories. Washing your solids down with liquids does not work either. Overdoing liquid calories between meals will result in a failure of the band to restrict. This is why an adjustment cannot fix the things you must do to assist the tool to its best performance.

Goal Weight Attained

Throughout this process, reaching the goal is the most rewarding moment for any patient. To make your goal reachable, your expectations have to be realistic. It is not realistic to say at age 60 you are going to get back to what you weighed at 19. Do any of us? Very few ever get down to that level of former weight and if they do, they tend to look older and drawn. Being realistic about that which is attainable will help you reach a more logical goal. Some people will challenge this and actually reach their desired weight; it has happened with patients. If you strive for perfection and do everything and anything necessary to reach it, YOU WILL SUCCEED!

On the other hand, if you depend on the band to do it for you, the probability is that the weight goal you aimed for will not be reached. Most patients fall close to their target and, after stabilizing, they fluctuate 10 pounds from that weight.

Keeping the Weight Off

Once you are at a stable weight, you need to determine if that is the weight with which you are comfortable. If not, you will have to try harder to reduce the weight that you most desire.

If you have arrived at your goal or ideal weight, your new goal will be keeping that weight stable. The most effective way to do this is by rewarding yourself for a job well done. You have reached your weight-loss goal successfully and should enjoy every minute of it. Your reward is flexibility and giving yourself a vacation with food. Choose one day out of the week that you can divert somewhat from the diet guidelines; call this the free food day. This means that, once a week, you eat whatever you want that you feel you can comfortably hold. You've earned it. The band will still limit your ability to over-eat, but whatever amount of calories you eat that free day of the week will not be enough to sabotage the great success you may have already attained. This thought of rewarding yourself often furthers your appreciation of the new you.

A word of caution. It is very easy to stray off course, so if you are going to reward yourself with a free day, be sure that it is only one day a week and that you sincerely have earned it. This is sort of the honor system of eating.

Remember the quote about swerving all over the road? You still get there, but it takes more time. It's true with the LAP-BAND. You can follow the guidelines as much as possible and you will get there faster. Once you get there, you have earned the right to lead a normal life by really enjoying food and not being afraid of the after-effects. Though, you have to be sensible.

Another tip that can help you keep the weight off is learning what foods don't go down as well as before the band. Avoid them altogether. Some patients find themselves caught in a vicious cycle of solid food getting stuck, band getting too tight, not tolerating solids, switching to liquids, and not losing weight. Once they tolerate solids for a while, food gets stuck again and the cycle repeats itself. If you think you are caught in this cycle, stop and think of what it is that you are doing wrong. The culprit is usually one or more of the following:

- Not chewing thoroughly
- Eating too fast
- Swallowing a bigger bite
- Eating fibrous foods

And just by going back to the 10 guidelines for success, you will always find your answer.

There are other recommendations, such as eating sensibly and exercising, changing habits, and all the things we've mentioned up to this point.

Sports and Other Activities

No restrictions have been documented for patients with the LAP-BAND; actually, the contrary has been seen after weight loss. Strenuous physical activity sometimes can affect the area of the port. It is believed that something similar to a muscle strain can take place and may require rest and pain killers if it happens. This event is very rare and is related to sudden quick movements. We recommend warming up before any sport or strenuous activity. This usually avoids any lesions.

Travel

When traveling with the LAP-BAND, simple precautions must be taken. It is easy to get dehydrated, especially if your food intake is low and traveler's diarrhea is contracted. Other aggravating factors can be nausea and vomiting. It is recommended that patients travel with their anti-nausea and diarrhea medicine. It is also important to visit your surgeon first if you plan on traveling and you think your band may be too tight. Loosening the band is important, since a tight band can cause food dislodgement and that, in turn, can aggravate tightness resulting in total obstruction. You don't want to be caught on a plane or in the middle of a Safari with a problem and no experienced LAP-BAND doctor around to resolve it.

Airports

Metal detectors are not usually activated by LAP-BANDs, though some models do activate the detector.

Airplanes

Air travel is usually a pressurized environment and the LAP-BAND itself is not altered by this.

Scuba Diving

Again, this is also a pressurized environment but no major side effects have been seen after scuba diving and the LAP-BAND.

Medications

At this time, no medications have been proven to be detrimental to the LAP-BAND. Most people take over-the-counter medications and these have not been a problem with the band. All medications have certain precautions and side effects that should be observed, whether you have a LAP-BAND or not. So, if you use pain killers, cold medicine, allergy pills, etc., use caution and preferably take these medications under medical supervision.

If your medication has been prescribed by a physician, your doctor should mention precautions and side effects of the medications.

Steroids

Certain diseases like Autoimmune Diseases (Lupus, Crohn's Disease) require steroids during the active phase of the disease. Even though medication has been known to cause stomach ulcers, it has not been related to band erosions into the stomach. Again, it is important to observe all necessary precautions indicated by the prescribing physician.

Anti-Inflammatory Drugs

Certain diseases like arthritis, muscle and joint disease, etc., require this type of drug to control symptoms. These medications are very aggressive on the inner lining of the stomach. They can cause mild inflammation (gastritis) to ulceration of the mucosa and intestinal bleeding. All of these are complications related to the use of these medications. However, with the necessary precautions, their use is not contraindicated with the LAP-BAND.

Vitamins

Though LAP-BAND patients rarely experience malnourishment or vitamin deficiencies, most patients during and after reaching their weight-loss goal regularly take vitamin supplements. This is a good habit that promotes a healthier lifestyle for the new you. Multivitamins are preferable. Some liquid and even spray vitamins have become very popular with patients.

Fertility and Pregnancy with the Band

Fertility and the Band

In Europe, the LAP-BAND is often called "The Fertility Band," due to so many banded women becoming pregnant a year or so after being banded. Hormones are only one of the factors that determine infertility. When weight-loss happens, the result is:

- Hormonal balance
- Agility
- Sexual activity

It is highly recommended that patients having the LAP-BAND procedure not get pregnant for the first eighteen months to two years. Weight loss starts as soon as the LAP-BAND is placed.-Fertility increases with weight loss. You can understand then that, if precautions are not taken, a patient can get pregnant early on without reaching even half of their weight-loss goal. Once weight loss is interrupted with pregnancy, the momentum and drive that keeps the patient enthusiastic about the LAP-BAND is also lost. Picking up after the pregnancy is harder since it usually will be more than a year after the LAP-BAND was placed with no result. It is also important to mention that the environment where the baby develops is not as healthy as it would be if the patient looses their excess weight before getting pregnant.

Pregnancy with the LAP-BAND

There is much positive experience with pregnancy and the LAP-BAND. If the band has done its work and loss of excess weight has occurred, the mother and the baby will be better off during the pregnancy and delivery.

During the early stages of pregnancy, the presence of morning sickness may be a reason for band deflation. Violent vomiting can cause a band to slip. This is why it is better to be safe than sorry. Once the vomiting stage subsides, a careful re-inflation of the band can be performed.

Pregnancy and the LAP-BAND go well together. Most patients can last the whole pregnancy without band deflation. Symptoms such as reflux may require treatment with band deflation. Most patients will be well-nourished and will not need band deflation unless indicated by the obstetrician/gynecologist.

No other alterations have been documented with the LAP-BAND during pregnancy.

Remember: With the LAP-BAND you reach a new eating baseline that permits you to live a healthy slim life, even if you are pregnant.

The Future of Weight Loss

Obesity is a disease and is one that is more likely controlled than cured. Its causes are complex and, for the most part, create an imbalance between what is consumed and what is burned as fuel. Therefore, the LAP-BAND is recommended as a permanent device.

The future is promising, and with every new day comes hope of finding the magical drug, hormone, or gene therapy to abolish obesity.

In the meantime, the LAP-BAND is the best option to keep your excess weight off.

If we do find the magical drug, hormone, or gene therapy to abolish obesity, the band can be simply deactivated by deflation or even removed without residual alteration of the abdomen or its functions, basically putting everything back the way it was. In the meantime, you can benefit from the weight loss the LAP-BAND provides.

While patients should be in contact with their physicians fairly often in the first five years, they may reduce this to every year or so thereafter. By that time, living with the LAP-BAND will have long since become second nature. Visits to the doctor will be for routine checkups or to change restriction level.

The LAP-BAND device has been around for a decade, and physicians have amassed a great deal of clinical experience with it. A number of patients had this procedure 10 years ago and still have the band with no complications or adverse effects and enjoy the benefit of a slimmer body. Most likely, they will live with the implant the rest of their lives.

Someday in the future, the anthropologists may call this the era of bands and bones.

15

Troubleshooting the Band

It helps to know that there are issues that can be addressed and rectified with proper insight and help. I've listed some of the more common problems you may encounter with the LAP-BAND. If you have any of these issues and feel that you are struggling alone, get in touch with your doctor. Also chat with your support group. There are solutions to the problems.

After Surgery First Week

PROBLEM	PROBABLE CAUSE	SUGGESTED CORRECTIVE ACTION
Bloating	Excessive bed rest. Band acts as one-way valve.	Meds sometimes help. Walking and physical activity help.
Gas pains	Same as above plus	Avoid carbonated liquids.

	sipping carbonated liquids through a straw.	Walking and physical activity help.
Shoulder pain	Irritation from gas used in surgery. Same as above.	Painkillers prescribed by doctor.
Nausea	Related to anesthesia.	Antivomiting medication.
Vomiting (after full recovery from anesthesia)	Early solid-food intake. Intestinal infection.	Consult doctor immediately.
Coughing (fever and malaise present)	Anesthesia Cold Lung infection.	Consult doctor.
Wound redness If excessive, may be infection (swelling, pain warm to touch)	Wound's normal process of healing. May require antibiotics.	Consult doctor.
Wound open (called dehisence)	Reaction to suture material, liquid collection (seroma) or infection.	Call doctor. Keep clean. Keep covered.
Wound bleeding	Direct trauma to wound. Breakdown of suture material. Preexisting collection of blood.	Consult doctor. Keep clean. Keep covered. If active, keep pressure.
Wounds leaking	Probable seroma (collection of serous liquid) .	Consult doctor. Keep clean/covered.

Wound leaking pus	Probable infection.	Consult doctor. Keep clean/covered. Antibiotics
Painful port area	Direct trauma, serum, blood, or pus collection.	Consult doctor. May require drainage. Requires antibiotics.
Painful port area	Direct trauma. Inadvertent injury during sleep, walking, or activity.	Consult doctor. Heat pads 15 minutes every 4 hours. Painkillers/ anti-inflammatory.
Difficulty breathing	Existing disease. Lung collapse/infection.	Emergency Room. May require hospitalization.
Dizzy spells	Check blood sugar if diabetic. Other disease.	Liquid sugar. Consult doctor
Painful swallowing	Tight band, hyperactive esophagus.	Consult doctor. Medications help.
Acid reflux	Tight band, solid food Dislodgment. Vomiting resulting in swelling pouch.	Consult doctor. Acid blockers. Liquid diet. May require special studies(barium swallow).

Before Your First Fill, from Surgery to Two Months

PROBLEM	PROBABLE CAUSE	SUGGESTED CORRECTIVE ACTION
Hungry during liquid phase	Not enough liquid protein. Eating when others eat. Head Hunger.	Add protein shakes (week 3) Keep away from kitchen, restaurants, hot foods.

	Others eating.	Drink lots of water.
Hungry during solid phase	Too many carbs. Not enough protein. Eating mushy foods. Washing down with water.	Keep to solids. Eat three times a day. No liquids during meals.
No restriction during first 8 weeks	Band is not adjusted at this. It needs to heal in place.	Follow guidelines. Do not despair. Restriction will come with first fill.
Moderate restriction during first 8 weeks	Band may be snug. Swelling may persist.	Eat slowly. Follow guidelines.
Severe restriction during first 8 weeks	Band may be tight/ swelling. Prolonged liquid phase. Early band slippage.	Consult doctor— may be important. Time is virtue. Rule out band slippage (barium swallow).
Weakness	Very rare. Usually related to very tight bands or coexisting disease	Consult doctor and run tests.
Low weight loss	High caloric intake, not following guidelines.	Don't despair. Follow guidelines. Lower BMI patients lose less weight. Consult nutritionist.

After First Fill at 8 Weeks after Surgery to First 6 Months

PROBLEM	PROBABLE CAUSE	SUGGESTED CORRECTIVE ACTION
Too tight after fill	Too much fluid in band.	Remove fill partially.
Can't tolerate solids	Food dislodged in upper pouch.	May cause band slippage if band not deflated.
Constant vomiting	Band too tight. Upper pouch swollen. Band slippage.	Consult doctor. Studies may be necessary. Loosen band.
Food gets stuck frequently	Not chewing thoroughly. Eating too fast, too much, too big bites. Eating wrong foods.	Follow guidelines. Get support. Try different foods.
Tried suggestions; food still gets stuck	Band may be too tight.	Loosen band.
Reflux symptoms; heartburn	Pouch swollen because of frequent vomiting, PBing.	See doctor. Loosen band. Acid blockers. Liquid diet.
No weight-loss	Plateau, you may be losing sizes but not weight.	Weight loss will soon restart. Check guidelines. You may need fill.
Tolerating more solid food	Band is loose. Not eating real solid foods.	Get a fill. Follow guidelines.
Not getting	Band is loose.	Get fill.

full **with solids**	Foods not solid enough. Washing them down with water.	Follow guidelines.
Incisions **very hard**	Healing process.	Soft massage over incisions Keep waist and bra away from incisions. Don't poke at them.
Port area **very hard** **or swollen**	May be healing process. If painful, may be hurt inadvertently. If red and warm, may be infected.	See doctor. Rule out erosion. May require local treatment/antibiotics.
Port or tube **protruding** **under skin**	Port or tube migration. Port flipped.	See doctor. May require surgical revision.

This is meant to be a guide, but always seek medical attention and never leave anything unattended. ALWAYS CHECK WITH YOUR DOCTOR!

16

Frequently Asked Questions about the Band

These questions are the ones most often asked of LAP-BAND surgeons and their coordinators, or are asked on the various online LAP-BAND patient groups. See Chapter 11, which addresses frequently asked questions that are related to insurance, illegal discrimination based on weight, and other legal issues. This chapter will have certain redundant information, reiterating what is covered in other chapters.

Q. What is LAP-BAND surgery?
A. It has been called a physical intervention for behavior modification, for the LAP-BAND physically causes its recipient to modify his or her eating behavior.

LAP-BAND surgery is a minimally invasive procedure placing an adjustable gastric band around the upper part of the stomach to form a small gastric pouch, limiting the amount of food consumed. Customized through adjustments performed as needed after surgery, saline solution is injected with a small needle through the adjustment port that lies just underneath the abdominal skin and fat to accommodate your changing needs without further surgery. Long-term weight loss is similar to those of Gastric Bypass in five-year studies.

Q. Is the LAP-BAND approved in the United States?
A. Yes, after over a three-year trial period, it was approved for clinical use on June 5, 2001, by the Food and Drug Administration.

Q. Why the LAP-BAND rather than Gastric Bypass?
A. Far greater safety and with similar long-term results. With more than 150,000 performed worldwide, LAP-BAND surgery has been proven safe.

If less is fine, more is not necessarily better. This means that with the LAP-BAND, weight loss has equaled that of the Gastric Bypass, but with the benefits of a safer, gentler procedure. Recent studies have proven this fact. Now, numerous hospitals and centers in the United States are offering it, as well as other renowned centers around the world.

The adjustability is what gives the LAP-BAND that advantage. And because the stoma of LAP-BAND patients is adjusted, regaining of weight occurs less frequently; thus, failures are avoided.

Q. Is LAP-BAND surgery less effective than other weight-loss options?

A. LAP-BAND surgery is far more effective at producing weight loss than diet, exercise, drugs, and hypnosis by a factor of 15 or 20. LAP-BAND surgery is less effective in producing early weight loss compared to Gastric Bypass surgery. The weight loss is equaled after the first year. The main advantage of this is the quality of tissue that remains. It is no secret that rapid weight loss will produce very loose skin and folds.

Q. Do I qualify as a candidate for surgery?

A. To be considered for surgery in the Unites States, you must meet the following FDA guidelines:

- Are 100 pounds or more over ideal body weight or have a BMI of 40 or greater.
- And/or have a BMI greater than 35 with associated health problems related to obesity. These include hypertension, heart disease, high cholesterol level, diabetes, respiratory problems, gastro-esophageal reflux, stress, urinary incontinence, degenerative arthritis, and venous stasis disease/ ulcers.
- Have tried medically-supervised dieting to lose weight and have been unsuccessful at keeping it off.
- Be motivated to commit yourself to a change in your life.
- Not be suffering from other diseases that could have caused obesity, such as thyroid.
- Be between the ages of 18 and 60.

Q. How much weight can I expect to lose?

A. Studies around the world have determined that up to 70% of the excess weight is lost with the LAP-BAND. Our center has results similar to most centers around the world. A few centers in the United States have corroborated this fact.

A multi-country European study was conducted with 3,800 LAP-BAND patients. The mean percentage of excess weight loss at the three-year level was 73%. These results may vary due to the level of proper diet and exercise following surgery.

Q. How long has LAP-BAND surgery been performed?

A. The LAP-BAND was first placed in Huy, Belgium in September of 1993 by Dr. Mitiku Belachew. Soon after, it was introduced in 1993 in Australia, Europe, and Mexico. In the United States in June of 2001, the Food and Drug Administration approved the BioEnterics Band produced by INAMED Corporation for use in the United States. Surgeons in the U.S. have been proctored (trained to do the surgery) by surgeons from Europe, Australia, and Mexico, where the surgery has been done for more than a decade at the time of this writing.

Q. Why is the LAP-BAND not as popular as the Gastric Bypass?

A. LAP-BAND is very popular in Europe, Australia, and Mexico. It is actually the preferred weight-loss surgery, except in a few centers. In the United States, a three-year trial period had to be completed to approve the band for clinical use. Furthermore, every surgeon desiring to perform this procedure must undergo a strict training program and surgical proctoring before actually offering it.

Q. I have heard that when obese surgeons in the United States are considering weight-loss surgery for themselves, they have LAP-BAND surgery instead of Gastric Bypass. Is this true?
A. In a recent poll, when weight-loss surgeons were asked if given the need to have weight-loss surgery on themselves or their loved ones, the majority chose the LAP-BAND over any other procedure.

Q. Is the band permanent?
A. No. It can be removed, though very few ever are, there being no need to remove it. The band is designed to be a permanent tool in weight reduction. If the band is removed, the stomach will return to normal and food consumption generally increases. The patient often returns to his or her original weight and sometimes more.

      I have always said, in the future centuries, archeologists will be uncovering "bands and bones."

Q. How many types of bands are there?
A. Currently, there are six brands of adjustable gastric bands available worldwide:

- INAMED BioEnterics LAP-BAND System®
- MIDBand
- Swedish (Obtech) Band
- A.M.I. ® Soft Gastric Band

- Heliogast
- Gastrobelt

See Chapter 6 for detailed information. Only the INAMED product has been approved in the United States. The Swedish (Obtech) Band, also called a soft band since it does not have the hard outer shell, was in trials at the time this book was written, but FDA approval could not come before 2005.

Q. What is a soft band?
A. It is a band made from a material that is more pliable or flexible. It also means that the balloon is softer. The LAP-BAND has versions of hard and soft bands, though no clinical difference has been supported.

Q. Will the soft band become the most popular when approved by the FDA?
A. It depends on the ability of this new band to outperform the other two sizes. For the time being, its biggest advantage is for higher BMI patients; it is larger, therefore, it fits them better.

Q. Is it true that softer bands produce fewer complications, slippage, or erosion?
A. No study has proven that a certain type of band is better. All bands are foreign bodies. INAMED has perfected upon three things: 1) Biomedical device engineering: this means that the implant will function, not leak or deteriorate; 2) Training: every surgeon uses the same time-proven technique; 3) Follow-up: the longest follow-up studies on banding are on

the LAP-BAND System. Other band providers have designed implants that are softer, wider, and contain more volume, but none have proven to be more effective.

Because the LAP-BAND is a foreign body, the improved surgical technique now in use avoids these complications. The frequency of erosions is now very rare, but since the LAP-BAND is a foreign body, the risk, though minimal, will always be there.

Q. What are the different size bands?
A. The lengths of the INAMED LAP-BAND approved for use in the United States are either 9.75 centimeters or 10 centimeters. An 11-centimeter band is not available in the United States and is infrequently used worldwide. At the time of this printing, the new 13-centimeter band named the VG has been introduced. The capacity of the INAMED band is 4 cubic centimeters (4 cc) or milliliters (4 ml). The new VG has up to 10 cubic centimeters. (10 cc). Other brands have different fill volumes from 4 to 9 cubic centimeters.

Q. Do you place the VG during surgery now?
A. Certain centers have no access to the VG, and others are either using it selectively for larger patients or routinely on all patients.

Q. Will the band interfere if I need other types of surgery?
A. It depends on the type of surgery. If the desired operation affects the area near the band area, it may be done. The two typical operations that may be performed at the same time as the placement of the LAP-BAND are repair of a hiatal hernia

(hernia or rupture of the diaphragm at the place the esophagus passes through it) and cholecystectomy, more popularly called gallbladder removal. Many surgeons (including the author) often repair the hiatal hernia as part of the banding operation. Some may perform the cholesystectomy at the same time as a planned dual operation, if deemed necessary.

Q. Can I have another surgery performed at the time of my banding?
A. Yes. As mentioned in the previous answer, two typical procedures performed during banding are hiatal hernia repair and cholesystectomy. Hiatal hernia repair should be considered when a hiatal hernia is present, regardless if symptoms of reflux (heartburn) exist. The surgeon performing the LAP-BAND performs the hiatal repair if he considers it necessary.

Cholesystectomy is also considered if a patient has gallstones and has symptoms. Most surgeons will not perform a gallbladder removal if the patient is not symptomatic. The risks of performing this during LAP-BAND should not outweigh the benefits.

Other procedures may be performed such as inguinal hernia repair, umbilical hernia repair etc. They should be thoroughly discussed with your surgeon. Remember, the main reason you are having surgery is for weight loss, so the main procedure should be the LAP-BAND placement. All other procedures should be of secondary importance unless otherwise indicated by your treating surgeon.

Q. Is the surgery always done laparoscopically?
A. Almost all LAP-BAND surgeries are done laparoscopically, usually with five keyhole incisions varying from 5 milli-

meters to the largest being approximately 2 centimeters long. However, in rare cases, the surgery may need to be converted to the open approach. This should not be considered a complication. Surgeons will never hesitate to make a formal incision if needed. This is called a conversion from a laparoscopic to an open approach. Conversions are performed when the level of difficulty related to a higher BMI patient requires the change of approach. Conversions are also required in emergency situations, and we never hesitate to do so. Our main goal is to provide the safest surgery possible. And if a conversion is required, so be it.

A conversion typically will prolong the hospital stay by hours, and the relative complications to it are very low. This should also be fully discussed with your surgeon.

Q. Is the "open" surgery more dangerous than the laparoscopic approach?
A. All surgery has inherent risks. Open surgery has a longer recovery time and has more complications related to the incision. Open surgery is always considered as a viable and sometimes a lifesaving approach.

Q. Where are the incisions located?
A. Since all surgeries, surgeons, and patients are unique, most incisions will vary. The typical placement is five incisions around the higher part of the abdominal wall. They will vary in length from 5 to 12 millimeters and will vary in placement, depending on the patient. A wider incision is always used to accommodate the adjustment port.

Q. What preoperative tests are required?

A. Patients undergo a comprehensive set of evaluations to assist in performing safe and successful weight-loss surgery. Tests may include analysis of blood and urine, chest x-rays, cardiology, psychological/behavioral, respiratory function to determine lung capacity, and nutritional screening. Patients are checked for general health and for any conditions directly related to morbid obesity where surgery may provide benefit. For many, this may be a lifesaving procedure and require additional testing until the health status and risk factors are acceptable. It is wise to be patient.

Q. How long does the actual surgery take?

A. Surgery takes as long as needed. There are many variables affecting the length of the operation. The surgeon will let you know what to expect. On average, the procedure takes about an hour. In addition, time may be prolonged due to prep time before the surgery, outside, and inside the operating room, additional last-minute testing, etc. Repairing a hiatal hernia and other unexpected surgical findings can double or triple the standard length of the operation.

Q. What type of anesthesia is used?

A. General anesthesia is always used. This is the only way laparoscopic approach can be performed, especially in high-risk patients. Specifics of the anesthetic technique should be discussed with your surgical group, as different groups have different protocols.

Q. What is the recovery time?
A. Recovery time varies per patient. Usually patients are up and about a few hours after the procedure. Walking is highly encouraged after the procedure and assists in a shorter recovery time. Pain medication is administered, but abdominal tenderness, shoulder pain, and bloating may cause discomfort for some patients during early recovery. Discharge from the hospital generally occurs 12 to 48 hours after the procedure. Most patients can resume normal activities in 5 to 7 days, though many are back at nonphysical work in 3 days.

Q. What are these gas pains referred to by other patients?
A. Gas pains come from the CO_2 used to insufflate the abdomen (inflate it like a balloon so the surgeon has a good view of the organs). They are usually described as pains in the left shoulder and back, or pain felt when taking deep breaths. It is caused by the irritation the CO_2 creates in the inner lining of the abdominal cavity. It is controlled with common painkillers, such as Tylenol and Advil, and almost always disappears after the first 72 hours. Walking greatly helps diminish the discomfort.

Q. Are there any long-range effects from having gas pumped into my abdomen for the laparoscopic surgery?
A. No. The effects are temporary and usually are the result of the irritation described in the previous Question and Answer.

Q. Is bloating common?
A. Bloating occurs in a patient who has not had any food or water for a prolonged period of time, undergoes a surgical

procedure that insufflates and manipulates the abdominal cavity, and then is immobilized for a long period of time. Gas accumulates in the intestines, and diminished bowel movements further increase the bloating. This can be a source of discomfort and should be avoided by early and frequent walking after the surgery.

Q. What type of special diet is required following surgery?
A. After the surgery, the band needs to heal in place. Any solid food during the first three weeks could move the band from its position and create an early slip. This is why, for the first three weeks, liquids are indicated, starting by a first week of clear liquids, followed by a second week of full liquids, then a third week where liquid protein is added. See Chapter 9 for further information.

Q. What are mushy foods?
A. While scrambled eggs and tuna may sound like mushy food, they are actually solid food. You should keep away from true mushy foods, such as applesauce, soups, yogurt, mashed potatoes, cream of wheat, and cream of rice. These foods are not restricted by the band and can actually make you gain weight. After the third week, the patient is encouraged to eat solid foods.

Q. Will I be able to eat all types of food?
A. Again, different patients have different reactions, but with only a few exceptions, patients can eat or drink anything. Bread, spicy foods, and pasta are often cited as the exceptions. As to beverages, many banded patients have difficulty

with carbonated beverages such as beer and soft drinks. Some feel that the pouch is expanded by these drinks, though no evidence of such expansion has been produced. Since those with a LAP-BAND must take in a large amount of protein, they find that they have little room for complex carbohydrates like bread, pasta, rice, potatoes, sugar, ice cream, etc.

The true goal is to have the patient eating quality solid food, and eating a third of the original volume of intake.

Q. Why is protein so important?

A. The body needs a certain level of protein to maintain muscles (and also keep your hair production healthy). Protein has main functions in the body, structural and metabolic. This means that protein is the skeleton of the tissue. It is also involved in most of the chemical reactions that keep your body functioning.

Q. What do you mean by carbs craving carbs?

A. Carbohydrates (sugars) are easily digested, especially those that have been processed. The faster they are digested and go into your bloodstream, the greater the impact they will cause after they have been absorbed. You will feel hungry very soon after ingesting them, and the cycle begins again.

Q. Can I go on a low-carb diet?

A. Carbs are part of a balanced meal. With the LAP-BAND it is advisable to follow a balanced intake. It permits you to enjoy food in quality, but less in quantity.

Q. Will I be able to drink with meals?

A. It is highly recommended that you not drink immediately before a meal or within half an hour following the meal. This gives an opportunity for the pouch to fill and the nerves to signal a full feeling. The addition of fluids lubricates the food and it drains down the stoma more quickly.

Q. Will I be able to drink alcoholic beverages?

A. No, at least they are not recommended until you reach or near your goal weight. Alcoholic beverages will not irritate the band. They provide a rich, huge source of useless calories and they should be avoided. Since the patient is eating far less, a smaller amount of alcohol will result in intoxication. An occasional glass of wine or other alcoholic beverage is not considered harmful to weight loss.

Q. How much should I be able to eat per meal?

A. When you are appropriately filled, you should be eating approximately one third of what you formerly ingested. Figure it as about half the size of your fist. When you reach goal weight, your band may be adjusted to allow you to eat more, but you will not return to the former amounts.

Q. Will I still feel hungry all the time?

A. No. The LAP-BAND makes you eat less and feel full in two ways: first by reducing the capacity of your stomach, and second by increasing the time it takes food to get through the digestive system. When the pouch is filled with food, the nerves signal the body that it is full and hunger feelings are turned off. Food is slowly digested and trickles into the lower part of the stomach and then into the intestines. This gives a full, satisfied feeling for a longer period of time. If you follow the nutrition guidelines, when you choose your food and then chew it well, you should not feel hungry or deprived. LAP-BAND patients typically do not feel physical hunger for 6 to 8 hours following a meal.

Remember, there is physical hunger and there is food anxiety, also called head hunger. If you feel the urge to chew, get some sugarless gum. If you have the urge to swallow, drink some water or other non-caloric beverage such as iced tea.

Q. Should I have several small meals a day or three larger ones?
A. Larger is relative: Call it post-band normal, which as stated above is about a third of what you formerly ate. Since the object is to take in the smallest amount of food while avoiding hunger, three meals a day is ideal.

Q. Can vegetarians be banded?
A. Absolutely, though they must be very careful to make sure that they ingest enough protein.

Q. What about raw vegetables?
A. Caution should be taken when eating raw vegetables that have abundant fiber, since this can dislodge down the esophagus even with thorough chewing (Asparagus, broccoli, celery etc.).

Q. What happens if I eat too fast?
A. A LAP-BAND patient quickly learns to eat slowly because food must be chewed into tiny pieces or a piece will stick in

the stoma. A chunk of food too big for the stoma will be like a stone in an hourglass: nothing will pass through. This causes a very uncomfortable feeling of pressure, creating a large amount of thick saliva that LAP-BAND patients call slime. Then regurgitation takes place. This is commonly known as PBing.

Q. What is PBing?
A. As described in the question above, ingestion of a piece of food that will not pass through the stoma causes great discomfort, creating a thick saliva ("slime" and PBing), which is the need to regurgitate the contents of the stomach. This is not the typical forceful vomiting of the pre-band days, filled with chunks of food, but typically pinkish goo of half-digested food plus the offending chunk.

Q. Will the LAP-BAND cause heartburn?
A. Once in place, the LAP-BAND controls heartburn. It is actually considered as an anti-reflux procedure for most. A small percentage of LAP-BAND patients will experience some irritation and heartburn. The reason is usually swelling and inflammation at the pouch caused by excessive eating, PBing, or vomiting. When symptoms arise, you should immediately advise your doctor for treatment. The treatment is usually medications, diet modification, and band deflation. Remember, not treating this can lead to a severe complication and result in band removal.

Q. Will the LAP-BAND surgery cause constipation?
A. Yes, for some. Less food and water means fewer bowel movements. Some LAP-BAND patients find that they have

bowel movements only every three to six days. Drinking six to eight glasses of water a day or more will generally alleviate constipation problems. Fruits and sometimes medication may be required, but always consult your doctor. The lack of daily bowel movements is not a health problem.

Q. Will I need to take vitamin supplements?
A. Vitamin deficiency is not a usual problem with LAP-BAND patients. Most surgeons will recommend a daily supplement. The comparison is to Gastric Bypass surgery and other malabsorptive procedures, where since only a portion of food, vitamins, and medications are absorbed, vitamin supplements are critical and the dosages of vitamins have to be increased, monitored, and taken for life.

Q. Will I be able to drink carbonated beverages?
A. Once it was thought drinking carbonated beverages contributed to slippage, causing bloating, burping and discomfort. They should be avoided during the initial weight-loss period.

Q. What about swallowing my medications after surgery?
A. Larger pills should be split. Smaller ones should be swallowed with abundant water. Certain medications can be switched to a liquid form if available.

Q. Is it true that certain medications should not be taken with the band?
A. No, there is no evidence to suggest that. But there are medications that can inflame your esophagus and stomach.

The normal precautions for that certain type of drug should always be observed.

Q. What type of exercise is recommended after surgery?
A. As many receiving the LAP-BAND are severely obese, high-impact exercise is not advisable until the patient has lost enough weight to make it safe. Walking on streets or a treadmill, bicycling, and exercises that involve weights are recommended. The length of exercise is not as critical as the regularity.

Q. What is a fill?
A. The wonderful feature of the LAP-BAND is its adjustablity. The inner surface of the band contains a balloon that is connected by tubing to a reservoir called a port. The port is placed underneath the skin deep in the muscle tissue and is accessed with a fine needle. By injecting the port with saline solution, the inflatable part of the band fills like an inner tube and squeezes the stomach to make the stoma smaller. This is called a fill. Conversely, in case of pregnancy, severe illness, or upon reaching goal weight, the saline solution can be withdrawn to make the stoma larger. This is called an unfill or fill removal.

Q. What is an adjustment?
A. This is another name for a fill or fill removal.

Q. When do I need my first fill?
A. Most patients receive their first fill around six to eight weeks after the surgery.

Q. Why not have a fill right after the surgery?
A. The first fill is postponed exactly the time needed for the band to heal in place. At that time, three weeks have passed on liquids. Then we need you on solids to evaluate how much the band is truly restricting your food intake. This requires an additional three to five weeks. Not following these orders can jeopardize the band and your weight loss.

Q. How often will I need a fill?
A. The number of fills varies from patient to patient. Most patients receive from two to five fills during the first year. The right fill depends on you following the guidelines, especially eating solid foods. It also depends on if it is performed under x-ray guidance or not. This data is not published but has been our experience.

The ideal fill is that which permits you to eat solid food, a third of your pre-band intake. If you can eat less or more and are not losing weight, you may need a fill.

Q. Do I always need to have a fill with fluoroscopy?
A. Some surgeons do not use fluoroscopy for adjustments. The author believes that to be precise and to find the "sweet spot" faster, fluoroscopy is important.

Q. What does fluoroscopy entail?
A. A fluoroscope is a real-time x-ray machine, in which a low-power x-ray tube is connected to a TV monitor. The patient swallows a solution containing barium, which shows up white on the monitor. The physician inserts a needle into the port through the abdomen wall and then adjusts the amount of

saline in the inflatable portion of the band until the flow of barium into the stomach is ideal.

Q. Do fills hurt?
A. Like any injection, there is a tiny bit of pain, though because of its location in the abdomen, where there are few pain receptors, most patients hardly notice it.

Q. What is an overfill?
A. If too much saline solution is injected, the stoma is too small and will not permit enough food or fluid to go through the stoma.

Q. What can happen if I am overfilled?
A. A band that is too tight is dangerous. It can cause repetitive vomiting and food dislodging down the esophagus. In the worst case, one of these episodes can cause your band to slip. Fill removal should be immediately indicated.

Q. Where is the port located?
A. It can be located literally anywhere. Typically, it is located in the abdomen, placed three or four inches to the left of the navel and two or three inches above it. Some other areas are the high abdomen and sternum.

Q. What happens if my port "flips?" Can I still get a fill?
A. Port flips are not common, but when they do appear, the port can be coaxed into position for a fill either by touch or under x-ray guidance. Some ports may require minor surgery to reposition them.

Q. Will I be able to see or feel the port?
A. You may be able to feel it, but you can rarely see it. In the event of full weight-loss, some people may require minor surgical repositioning of the port, though this is a rare occurrence.

Q. Will anyone be able to tell I had the surgery?
A. It depends on the patient. Since the whole experience will last a couple of days, most people get back to their routine soon after that. It is the weight loss that typically gives you away, letting friends, colleagues, and relatives know by observation that you are losing a lot of weight.

Q. Should I tell anyone I had weight-loss surgery?
A. What you choose to tell them is up to you. Within a month or two after surgery, even casual acquaintances will notice that you have lost weight. Since as a LAP-BAND patient you will lose 50 to 250 pounds or even more, this change in your body will be dramatic and very noticeable. Most LAP-BAND patients do share with others that they have had LAP-BAND surgery. Some actually go out of their way to talk to obese friends, relatives, acquaintances, and even strangers to share their wonderful experience.

Q. What is emotional eating?
A. Emotional eating is eating—often in large quantities and generally comprising "comfort" or junk foods—in response to feelings instead of hunger. Experts estimate that 75% of overeating is caused by emotions.

Q. Will I experience depression after surgery?

A. It is rare after LAP-BAND surgery. In fact, the opposite is most common. Studies indicate that when a severely obese person's weight is reduced, their quality of life improves significantly in terms of life expectancy and happiness. They feel stronger, mentally and physically.

Q. What about dining out, what precautions should I take?

A. Depending on your restriction level, you may need to order off the kids' menu and sometimes limit yourself to appetizers. Use the "plate" tip in Chapter 9 to help you select the right entree.

Q. What happens when I reach my goal weight?

A. When the ideal weight is reached and your weight is stable, there is no need to change anything. Some patients will consider that it will be time for an unfill, for some or all of the saline solution in the band to be removed until a new "sweet spot" is found where the weight will not increase or decrease. It is extremely rare for a person with a LAP-BAND to have it removed after reaching goal weight. This is a challenge to prove that your habits have become a lifestyle, a way of life.

Q. What are the risks of LAP-BAND surgery?
A. Laparoscopic banding involves the least risk of all surgeries performed under anesthesia. It is ten times safer than any other weight-loss procedure. The LAP-BAND placement is still considered major surgery and has inherent risks. In addition, obesity also contributes to these risks. All of the risks should be discussed with your surgical group prior to surgery. The most common surgical risks depend on the existence of major disease at the time of surgery. When no other disease is present, temporary early obstruction after the LAP-BAND placement can develop and is discussed in the appropriate chapter. Other complications include partial lung collapse, collection of serous liquid at the incisions, infection, etc.

Most of these are rare and simple to treat. Complications with diabetes causing high blood sugar can develop after the procedure. Heart and lung complications may also develop when severe disease is present. Most of these are controlled before the surgery to avoid the risks. Severe complications can develop during the procedure (gastric or esophageal perforation) and after (blood clot formation with embolism), even death. Every risk is assessed and controlled before surgery. This is why the preoperative evaluation and treatment are important. In medicine, the benefits should outweigh the risks, and the LAP-BAND is a great example of this.

Q. What about pregnancy?
A. Obesity causes infertility. Weight loss causes fertility. This means that once the weight loss starts, you may get pregnant easily. We recommend postponing pregnancy for twelve to eighteen months following the procedure when weight loss is the most substantial. The more weight loss experienced be-

fore pregnancy, the healthier the mother and child will be. Weight loss prior to conception also reduces the risk of gestational diabetes. Once pregnant, women require more extensive nutritional support. The LAP-BAND is easily adjustable to meet those needs. Also, banded women have no problem breastfeeding.

Q. Will I need plastic surgery after my weight-loss?
A. For some, plastic surgery will be desirable; for others, it will be necessary. Once weight loss is evident, loose skin will appear. Whether the skin contracts to fit the smaller body depends on genes, the age of the patient, and the amount of weight lost, even the type of skin. A typical patient having plastic surgery after LAP-BAND surgery will have lost more than 100 pounds and will choose a tummy tuck. Other areas that may require surgery include arms, legs, lower torso, back, buttocks, breasts, neck, and face.

Q. Where can I go to have plastic surgery done, and what type of surgeon does this?
A. Loose skin may appear after weight loss. The main areas affected are the abdomen, chest, thighs, arms, legs, neck, and face. The body recontouring and "lift" is performed by Plastic and Reconstructive surgeons, who are now considered specialty surgeons because of the degree of technical difficulty involved.

Q. How much does LAP-BAND surgery cost?
A. In the United States, the total cost of LAP-BAND surgery—including all hospital charges and doctor fees, but ex-

cluding fills and pre-operative tests—ranges from $15,000 to $30,000.

Q. Is the cost of LAP-BAND surgery covered by insurance?
A. A disappointing percentage of people covered by insurance are covered for LAP-BAND surgery; though, at the writing of this book, approximately one-quarter of insurance companies, HMOs, and PPOs do cover some LAP-BANDs while they cover more Gastric Bypass procedures. Insurers use the excuse that the LAP-BAND surgery is "experimental," despite the LAP-BAND being approved by the U.S. Food and Drug Administration in June of 2001. See Chapter 11.

Q. What should I do if my insurer refuses to cover LAP-BAND surgery?
A. See Chapter 11 of this book on what to do. You may need assistance in appealing the denial by your insurer. Check the web site: www.obesitylaw.com to find attorneys specializing in helping people appeal their denial by insurers. Walter Lindstrom of Obesity Law & Advocacy Center in San Diego is one.

Q. Is the cost of the surgery tax-deductible?
A. Medical expenses are deductible, but it is necessary to itemize. The tax deduction for medical expenses is the amount greater than 7.5% of your adjusted gross income. This includes expenses incurred outside of the United States. Check with your tax adviser, accountant, or IRS publications for the latest and most accurate information on deductibility.

Q. If I self-pay, what payment methods are available?
A. For surgeons in Europe and Mexico, the payment is usually made via wire transfer and/or by cashier's check prior to or on the day of surgery. Credit cards and financing are also available by the more established centers.

Q. What if I have a complication after surgery and my surgeon is in a different country?
A. Many hospitals are now LAP-BAND friendly, having passed the required training, including surgeons and their staff. Any hospital that is referred by the INAMED website is qualified to handle any such issue. Emergencies with the LAP-BAND are quite rare.

Q. What is the complication rate?
A. The rate of complications has drastically decreased in the last decade, as experience with the procedure increases and the bands are continually improved. At this moment, overall complications are less than 5%. Most of these are such conditions as partial lung collapse, wound infection, dehiscence (opening of a wound), etc. The major complications are not life-threatening and are below 2%.

Q. Are there drugs I must avoid?
A. Anti-inflammatory agents, such as aspirin, should be used with caution, but there is NO data to support they contribute to an increased risk of band erosion.

Q. Where can I find an experienced LAP-BAND surgeon?
A. The INAMED website http://www.INAMED.com/ has a surgeon locator for the United States. The Official Mexican INAMED website is www.mecachrome-medical.com. This site will also assist you.

Q. Where do I check my surgeon's credentials and reputation?
A. Most bariatric surgeons are members of their National Society of Bariatric Surgery, also members of International Societies such as IFSO (International Federation for the Surgery of Obesity). They may also belong to various other distinctions such as being Fellows of the American College of Surgeons (the letters FACS after MD).
Contacting other patients that have had the procedure at that given center will also be of value. Contacting the doctor's office for an appointment or interview is also a good idea.

Q. Could I fly directly after surgery?
A. Recovery to the point where taking a flight is advisable usually takes 24 hours, and some patients with more complicated problems would be wise to plan on an additional 48 hours. Some very high-risk patients should plan to stay up to a week. Consult your surgeon for recommendations on travel schedule.

Q. My surgery date is almost here and I am scared and nervous. Is this normal?
A. Most LAP-BAND candidates do extensive research on the various websites and online groups sites. They soon find out

that just about every pre-band person is scared and nervous, especially those who go out of the country for surgery. They also soon find out that these same patients report a few weeks after their surgeries that their fright and anxiety soon disappeared once the surgical procedure was over and they recovered from it.

Q. Will I feel weak after the LAP-BAND, the low-caloric intake, and so much weight loss?
A. No. It is impressive how people after losing a substantial amount of weight feel healthier and stronger. After having toted around 100 pounds or so of excess weight, it is mostly liberating.

Q. Will I be sick a lot after the operation?
A. The reverse is almost always true. You will be sick much less than before the operation.

Q. What are the possible major complications?
A. There are two: slippage and erosion. Slippage is the result of a stomach that slips through the band proximally. Vomiting can lead to slippage, so it should be avoided at all costs. Erosion is natural to any foreign body implanted in you. This happens when the band rubs on the stomach and eventually wears a hole in the stomach. Slippage and erosion are extremely rare. As experience increases, complications decrease drastically.

Q. How much weight should I expect to lose?
A. Though it varies from patient to patient, 30% excess weight loss during the first 3 months, 40% during the next 6 months, and 60% at 8 to 12 months.

Q. What is self-sabotage?
A. Self-sabotage is when banded people ingest too many calories by several means:
- Eating all day and night, rather than three solid meals.
- Eating high-carbohydrate foods. Ice cream and candy, for example, slip right through the band.
- Eating mushy foods.
- Drinking high-caloric beverages, such as milkshakes, whiskey, and beer.
- Washing down solid food with water.
- Not eating three times a day.
- Not getting band adjustment promptly.

Q. Does the LAP-BAND require frequent visits to my doctor after surgery?
A. Regular follow-ups with your doctor are a normal a part of the LAP-BAND experience. The doctor will define the schedule, based on regular telephone or email contact. Most patients will have success just by having the necessary fills at the precise time.

Q. Does the LAP-BAND limit any physical activity?
A. No. The LAP-BAND does not hamper physical activity, including aerobics, stretching, and strenuous exercise. Air travel and SCUBA diving present no problems.

Q. Do I have to be careful with the port just underneath my skin?

A. No special care need be taken. It is placed under the skin in the abdominal wall, and once the incisions have healed, it should not cause discomfort or limit any physical exercise. Early versions of the LAP-BAND sometimes had problems with the detachment of the hose between the band and the port. This problem has been resolved. If you feel persistent discomfort in the port area, talk to your doctor.

Q. Is it true that the LAP-BAND seems tighter in the morning?

A. This is fairly common. Sometimes solids are not tolerated during the morning hours. This can be resolved by "opening" your band with a couple of glasses of water. Some women have also reported that the LAP-BAND may feel tighter during menses.

Q. I had a Gastric Bypass five years ago and I am gaining my weight back slowly. Can I be banded?

A. While not every person who has had a Gastric Bypass can be banded, a large percentage can. Those who have gone through this report that they are extremely pleased with the results, that they are losing the weight they gained back. Very few LAP-BAND surgeons have experience with this operation, which is significantly more complex than a first-time LAP-BAND surgery. If you are in this situation, do a great deal of research to find a doctor who has done the operation before with excellent results. We discuss this in the appropriate chapter.

Q. Do men lose weight faster than women after banding?

A. Generally, yes. Men report a much smoother recovery period and have more rapid weight loss. I believe that this is because men tend to have a pattern of larger meals, which are not possible after banding, while many women have an eating pattern of ingesting small amounts during the day.

17

Their Success Stories

There have been some marvelous changes in the lives of many of my patients; most have succeeded in losing the extra weight, and yet a very few have failed to adhere to the guideline that I have clearly spelled out. Consequently, they have not lost their desired weight as have those depicted here in these very touching, dramatic stories on their journey to slimmer, more attractive bodies.

Please take the time to read their stories. You will not only gain a greater appreciation of the LAP-BAND, but you will also be inspired to follow their excellent example for losing weight.

Here they are—enjoy!

My Life Changed Completely

by

Cynthia P. Jones

"I'm forty-one years old. I was fat for about twenty-nine years. It doesn't matter why I got fat: we all have our reasons. What matters most is that I wanted to be invisible. It has always amazed me how a large person can be invisible. But I was! Of course, I went through periods of time where I wanted to be thin and I would try some diet and have success, but I would always gain the original weight back, plus a lot more. By the time I was 36, I weighed 340 pounds. In February of 1999, I gave up. I decided that God wanted me to be fat. I would never get married, never have children, and never have a life. I figured I had about ten more years on this planet and then I would die of congestive heart failure, hopefully in my sleep. This was between God and me. I told no one.

About one week after I had made this decision, my sister called and told me of a girl named Brandi who lost weight surgically, but not with the bypass surgery procedure. She quickly gave me her number and got off the phone. (You see, we didn't talk about weight in my family. It was sort of the big old elephant in the middle of the room that everyone would step around.)

My family is all of normal size. I was the only 'big' one. Every once in a while I got the 'You have such a beautiful face; if only you would lose the weight.' This would always send me into tears. Well, I called Brandi, and that very night I went to her apartment to see her. Here was this tiny girl who told me that she had just finished eating ice cream and chips, showing me a picture of herself at over 300 pounds. Ice cream and chips? This was for me! Within 24 hours, I was in New Orleans at Dr. Louis Martin's office. This was during the FDA trials and I had to jump through a few hoops in order to become one of the qualified patients. I passed all the tests and was given my band and a new life on March 29, 1999.

Now many people do quite a bit of research before one decides to get a band. I operated on faith alone. Sure, I listened to what the doctor told me, but all I knew was that this was my last chance. Right after I had surgery, Brandi got married and moved to Baltimore. I did not know of anyone else in Dallas that had the band. Good or bad, I was going through this adventure alone. What an adventure it has been!

The surgery experience went well. At first I didn't want anyone to know. After all, I was a failure; I couldn't 'eat less and exercise more.' I had to have surgery to get healthy. Well, that lasted about a week. Then I realized that I wasn't a failure: I was taking control of my life. I was doing something positive. I was SAVING my life! So, I told everyone! That led to my family and friends watching every morsel I put into my mouth, marveling at how little I could eat and not be hungry. When I got the 'deer in the headlights' look due to something being stuck and asked to be excused, someone always would ask, 'Are you going to throw up?' I no longer can go to the bathroom during a meal to even wash my hands without the 'throw up' comment.

I spent the adjustment phase circling the kitchen like a shark. I would walk in and open the fridge, realize I wasn't hungry, and leave. About thirty minutes later, I would do the same thing. Eating out was an event. A few bites into the meal, I was full. I would bring everything home. My refrigerator was a sea of white cartons. Of course once you have eaten the same thing four times, you don't really want it. Now I order a small portion or just leave it there. I am a great date! My friends and the guys I go out with get to have a meal and a half! The worst problem I experience now is on several occasions I have had chefs come out of the kitchen and ask what was wrong with the meal. Argh! I have to explain the band in order to keep their feelings from being hurt!

I had a ton of energy after dropping just a few pounds! I proceeded to needlepoint an entire Christmas stocking for my mother, and I even started cleaning my house. At one point, I had a toothbrush on the baseboards! Anything to keep busy and wrangle in some of this extra energy I had. No one really noticed I had lost much of anything until I had lost about 60 pounds. Then all of the sudden my clothes were loose, my face was thinner, and my body had started to change. This was around October of 1999. Of course, I still saw the 340-pound woman staring me back in the mirror. This prompted me to call Dr. Martin and request an appointment with him for my next fill. Everything was going well for me, but I thought I was going crazy! Dr. Martin explained that this was very normal and quickly put me on anti-depressants. He also prescribed three twenty-minute back massages a week! Love that man.

What I can tell you now is that the old Cynthia was in the process of dying; the new Cynthia was beginning to emerge. I didn't know what to make of the new me, and at the same time, I was mourning the old me. As the layers of fat were leaving my body, there was no place for me to hide. Suddenly, my clients were annoying me. I was a travel agent to a very wealthy, high-maintenance clientele. I became frustrated with their requests. The manager of the agency where I rented my desk had an extremely short temper with me. I couldn't understand what was going on. So, I sought the help of a therapist. Through discussing this matter with him, I realized that I was no longer a human doormat, and I had begun to stand up for myself. I had self-esteem! Well, my clients and coworkers, who were used to wiping their feet on my face, just didn't know what to make of this. I knew at that moment that my time in the travel business would be short-lived, and I began to look for someone to purchase my client list. Changes happen when you change your life. Please, don't be afraid to go and talk to someone about it. Jobs change, marriages and relationships begin and end, and some new friends enter your life as well as old friends leave your life. This is all part of change. Please, don't be afraid of it, but embrace it!

In late January of 2000, my body shifted whilst I was on a trip in Thailand. All of a sudden, I had a neck! I found some long lost friends, my collarbones! One year after the surgery, 120 pounds were gone from my life forever! Ok, we all have lost weight and had success, only to gain it all back. I was so scared that the same thing would happen with the band. This was too good to be true. I was waiting for the other shoe to drop. To test myself, I decided not to get a fill for a while and see if I would balloon back up to my original weight.

During my non-tight months, I decided it was time to do something about my breasts. They were huge cow udders! So, in May of 2000, I went under the knife for a breast lift and reduction performed by Dr. David Liland. I went from a saggy DD to a perky B! To be honest, it was more like a buh. But, hey, they were perky and I could walk around in a T-shirt without a bra and not look like I was smuggling melons! I also started exercising. I had sat on my butt for the first year and to be completely honest with you, that is my biggest regret! I started turning the jiggle into toned muscle. After losing over 100 pounds, I had a huge pannus or apron. It got hard to exercise with a girdle on in Texas heat. Time for the first tummy tuck! Before I went under the knife for a second time, I finally got another fill. Miracles of miracles, I had stayed within one or two pounds the whole time I was not on a tight fill! This was the real deal! I really was going to get thin! It was within reach!

Around Thanksgiving of 2000, I had ten pounds of skin removed from my lower abdomen. I was told this would be an extremely painful operation. Well, let me tell you, the pain was minimal. I woke up from surgery and could look down and see, as a friend lovingly put it, 'my hey nane nane.' Believe me, there was only joy! My advice to people considering a tummy tuck: Don't be afraid of the pain. It isn't like a tummy tuck for someone who has a little pooch. Everyone who has had one since has told me that I was the only one who said the pain wouldn't be bad, and I was right!

Three wonderful things happened after my lower tummy tuck. First, I found a buyer for my business and started all the legalities that come with selling a business. Next, I began to be noticed by the opposite sex; of course, I will get into that in a minute. Finally, I found out that there were other people that live in the DFW area who were banded. They had gone to Mexico. I no longer had to go through this alone!

Now, don't get me wrong. I could not ask for more supportive family or friends. My sister alone is someone who I credit for saving my life. She has been my biggest cheerleader! Oh, but to have some people that have been through the same experience. To bounce questions off them, to find out if they were going through the same changes—that was heaven! These people—Ester, Nelda, Amanda, and Katie— immediately became family to me. So many more have joined the ranks. I tell patients when they wake up from surgery, 'Welcome to Bandlandia,' as now they are part of an elite group of people that have an implant that will save their lives! It was a blessing to find them, and I am always thrilled to meet a newly banded person.

By March of 2001, I had sold my business and was ready to have my upper tummy tuck. Now, for most of you, one tummy tuck would suffice, but my plastic surgeon was concerned because I had a lovely 13-inch scar on my right side due to a gallbladder operation in 1986. So, off to operation number three. This was a dual operation, as my gynecologist found numerous tumors in my uterus and they, along with my right ovary, had to be removed and my uterus rebuilt. This was the result of my being too scared to get yearly checkups because I was so fat and embarrassed. Please, don't be afraid of your weight to get these things checked out. Luckily, my left ovary is intact and has loads of follicles! I can reproduce! Once again, the shape of the new body alleviated most of the pain.

By now I was a size 12 to 14. I was thrilled! I could go into any store I wanted and buy something that fit! No longer would I EVER have to step foot into Lane Bryant again! (Actually, my secret goal is to put Lane Bryant out of business.) By now, I was exercising almost every day. I could have cared less if I ever reached my goal weight! My trainer reminded me ever so gently that I wasn't supposed to be a 12 to 14; my body shape was to be smaller. He gave me the encouragement and the slap I needed to finish what I had set out to do. I no longer had to go to New Orleans for fills, as I had found a doctor in Dallas who knew of the band and administered fills. We immediately hit it off.

While selling my business and considering what I wanted to do with my life, the same answer kept popping into my head: I wanted to help people get the band. I knew at some point the band would become legal in the U.S., and then there would be a job for me. In the meantime, I continued to get to know as many banded folks online and in the Dallas area as I could. I kept experiencing shifts in my body. Not so much weight loss, but one day I would go to bed with a pair of pants that fit, and the next day they would be too big! My body was compacting. This to me is the strangest yet the most beautiful thing about the band. The LAP-BAND became FDA approved in the U.S. on June 5, 2001.

In March of 2002, I was offered a job to work as patient advocate for a company that helps people in getting the band. I had my final plastic surgery in April. Dr. Liland did my arms and thighs and a revision on the tummy tucks, and with guidance from Dr. Rodolfo Sanchez, he moved my port. Following this surgery for the first time, I could look in the mirror and no longer see the 340-pound girl, but actually a thin woman with a flat stomach and thighs that don't touch! My clothing size had become a 4 to 6. The first time I tried on size 4 jeans that fit, I kept making the salesgirl go and get me other pairs, as I kept thinking they were mismarked! I could wear high heels and not be in pain! I could tie my shoes with the laces straight and not to the side as they were before. You know what I mean, the art of trying to tie your shoes when you are big!

There is a shop in Dallas called Tootsies. For years I handled their travel account. I always loved their clothes, but, of course, they don't carry a size 28. Finally, I could walk in there and buy something. The salespeople used to laugh at me as I would grab the largest size and pray that it would fit. Of course, by now I was thinner, and a 12 was just too big. They would giggle as I walked back out and grabbed the 10, snicker some more as I came back out for the 8, and finally howl when I would again return for the 6. One of the salespeople, Adam, took pity on me and told me to just call him when I was coming in and he would pull the correct size for me from now on. This man has a client for life!

I would like to mention the body dysmorphia that many of you will go through during your weight loss. It took three years, over 200 pounds, and several plastic surgeries for me to finally see in the mirror what everyone else saw. Each morning, I am still amazed when I look in the mirror and see a thin me staring back. I have even turned around to look for the real me! Shopping has become one of my favorite activities. Today, I counsel patients to hold off as long as possible to buy nice clothes. Get the cheap stuff until you have hit your goal, and then buy the expensive clothes. I couldn't wait and, therefore, the Salvation Army has made a mint off of reselling the nice clothes I bought.

Now, you were wondering when I would get to the opposite sex, weren't you? Dating is new for me and will be new for you as you enter into the visible world. To be noticed by men is shocking and quite scary at first. I can still remember the first time a guy checked me out. It is one of those frozen moments. Silly me, I had to ask my friend if that guy was looking at me! I went on many dates with complete creeps for quite awhile, just to get into the groove of it all. I have made up for all those years of non-dating or being with total abusive losers in one year. I could relate some stories, but hey, you want to know about the band—not horror stories. I will tell you the latest winner. I met this guy for drinks, but he did not buy me one. Instead, he said that he thought I was hot and wanted to see if we were sexually compatible before we got to know each other. Good lord, the lines I have heard! The running joke around the office is how many dates does Cynthia have this week? The most I have done was six, but that was exhausting! I have met some wonderful men, too. Now I have the confidence to stand up for myself, and know I don't have to accept the first offer that comes my way!

I created Bandlandia because I saw a definite need on getting people from big to little and all that it entails. I get to help people become healthy and enjoy life. Four years ago, my life was hopeless. Now it is full of hope! I have a dream job, and the possibility of getting married and having children is within reach. I have self-confidence; I have learned to love myself; and hey, I look good! People that see me for the first time since I lost weight have said, 'Oh my gosh, Cynthia, you have lost a person...' I usually reply, 'No, I found one.'

At Christmas, my mother gave me a hand towel that now hangs in my office. It says, 'What the caterpillar thought was the end of life, the butterfly realized was just the beginning.' Every person who has had weight-loss surgery is a butterfly on a wonderful adventure. Enjoy every step of the way, the good and the bad, because now you HAVE a life. And a healthy one at that! Thank you for your time!"
Cynthia P. Jones

Why I Had LAP-BAND
by
Lee Grossbard, M.D.
LAP-BAND Surgeon and Patient

"I was 50 years old and morbidly obese. At 5 feet 5 inches short (vertically challenged when you are obese), I weighed 265 pounds. This yielded a BMI of over 44. Like most morbidly obese patients, the search was on. All morbidly obese patients use the Internet. We are the most adapted to use technology to our advantage. It does not take long to learn the advantages and disadvantages of all of the available remedies, once the decision to do something is made.

That initial decision may take many years for most patients, but it seems that the decision is now being made easier for most. I weighed about 150 pounds when I graduated from high school. The usual college freshman diet and my own weight fluctuated around 175 pounds for the next couple of years. Gradually, over the next five years, my weight got up to 191 pounds. Marriage was on the horizon and weight loss to fit into the tuxedo was desirable. A pickle diet along with salad was utilized. A marriage-date weight of 158 pounds was reached with time to spare. Over the next two and one-half decades, the weight vacillated, and eventually the zenith of 265 pounds was realized. How does the patient make the decision to finally have surgery for a chronic problem that we are taught is self-induced?

Is it self-induced?

Was it genetic?

But I tried to lose weight so many times. I've lost 50 pounds at least ten times in the last ten years. I can do it again. Can't I? Should I lose the weight medically or surgically?

Do they have a discount for the baker's dozen with Weight Watchers?

Why won't the FDA allow Fen-Phen back on the market?

All of these questions are valid for the obese patient. I looked to the Internet for some of the answers. The Internet leads to many sites that are informative; however, many sites are filled with nonsense and misinformation. In fact, the worst part of the Internet resources that obese people are confronted with is disinformation.

There exists on the Internet the utterly amazing utility to sell something. Anything and everything is for sale on the Internet. Sponsored sites for weight loss include sales for high-protein shakes that have more calories per cubic centimeter than Vivonex.

Once the decision to have surgery is made by the patient, the next question is what type of surgery?

As we all know, there is no unanimity on this question. For some patients who do their own research, this is an easy question to answer. Most prospective patients who are Internet savvy know more about the surgical options and where they are available than most surgeons would ever dream of.

Do I stay in the United States or do I go abroad?

If I go outside of the U.S., do I go to Mexico, Australia, or Europe?

All of these questions went through my mind, as I am sure they have gone through most patients' minds. But what about the primary question, will it be bypass or LAP-BAND?

The most confusing issue to the majority of patients appears to be what exactly a bypass is. The terminology that is used includes Gastric Bypass, mini-gastric bypass, open gastric bypass, Roux-en-Y bypass, Lap Roux-en-Y bypass, RNY, Lap RNY, BPD, duodenal switch, long limb RNY, etc. All of this confuses the majority of patients.

Through the haze that surgeons create that makes them stand out as individuals, the patient eventually understands the differences between metabolic, restrictive, and combined procedures.

Most patients do not ever need a purely metabolic procedure. If by some chance they are in the super obese category and have met other criteria, then they migrate towards the metabolic procedures and the centers that tend to do the largest loads of these procedures. The older procedures that were restrictive in nature are generally not utilized today. Though there still exists pockets of surgeons performing VBG, vertical banded gastroplasty, and nonadjustable bands, they are not numerous and are relatively difficult for patients to find. The ability to perform a laparoscopic VBG is not readily available to most surgeons and patients. Well, at this point, the patient understands that their choice usually comes down to a bypass or a LAP-BAND.

This past year has seen an enormous growth in the number of bariatric centers, surgeons, and options. Most patients are not referred by another physician to the bariatric surgeon. Patients garner information from the Internet, other patients, and advertising much more readily than from surgeons and other physicians. The one possible exception to this is the medical bariatric specialist.

These doctors come in two forms, the entrepreneurial specialist and the altruistic physician who wants to help cure obesity. If the physicians belong to the latter group, then they usually will work with their patients for a set period of time before calling for the aid of the bariatric surgeon. Very aggressive advertising by some bariatric programs has turned many patients off. What then is the right amount?

We can usually say what is 'over the top' but have difficulty in stating what the correct amount is. It appears that the university programs tend not to advertise to the general public as much as the private sector. If this is true, then why are the majority of patients being done where they are paying for the advertising?

Once the patient has made a decision to attend a seminar, he or she has choices: who teaches the seminar, what procedure and/or a procedure are offered, and is there a bait-and-switch going on?

All are valid and cogent questions asked by many patients. The bypass procedure is well-documented in the literature for over 25 years. Its efficacy is without question even by the most diehard LAP-BAND surgeons. We patients are all able to understand what the mortality and morbidity figures for procedures mean. The problem is what do we know about the individual surgeons?

I, for one, have always heard bariatric surgeons state that their mortality rates are well below 0.5%. However, when groups such as SAGES and the ASBS regularly state that the real mortality figures are much higher, who does the patient believe?

There is no doubt that there exists an elite group of surgeons in both private and academic practice that truly achieve a leak rate of around 2% and a mortality rate of about 1/2%. But these programs are the exception and not the norm. At a university program that states a 1/2 percent mortality rate where there are three deaths within a two-week period, how can the director still claim a 1/2 percent mortality rate?

Patients do come to the conclusion that the adjustable bands are a safer procedure than a bypass. It really does not take a large amount of intuition for most to reach this conclusion. The next step for many patients is to decide which adjustable band to proceed with. Currently, in the United States the only approved band is the LAP-BAND made by INAMED. The Swedish band is to be tested and marketed by

Ethicon, a Johnson & Johnson subsidiary, but is still in the A trials at the time this is written.

Also to be considered by some patients are the other variants of adjustable bands that are available in Europe and Latin America. It is usually during this period of Internet exploration that some patients hear of the nonadjustable bands that have been performed in the U.S. for over two decades. A new bifurcation in the tree of choices springs up that also confuses the primary issue: what surgical procedure is best? The long-term data for nonadjustable banding in the U.S. is difficult to come by. There are many testimonials from all over the U.S. about the procedure, but scientific data is not obtainable. Curiously, many of the testimonials are not very flattering. Where do I get my LAP-BAND done?

There are currently over 400 U.S. surgeons that have taken the FDA-approved courses for the LAP-BAND. There are about 200+ surgeons that have been proctored in the U.S. There are about 170 that are active LAP-BAND surgeons. What about going to Mexico where the cost is less?

Is it that much less?

Yes, it is. However, with the IRS write-off, is it really less?

Not really! The primary reason today for Americans to go to Mexico is for a particular surgeon with much larger experience and numbers of cases and for those who are refused the operation in the United States. The reasons for refusal in the U.S. are mainly FDA requirements. We are starting to see larger and larger numbers of patients that go out of the U.S. because they want the LAP-BAND and their BMI is less than the requisite 35 for operation in the U.S. Also, patients below the age of eighteen are starting to make their appearance in other countries because of the FDA rules. What about American surgeons going outside the U.S. to meet their patients' requests for LAP-BAND surgery?

This, too, has the potential of increasing in number in the near future. Many American surgeons tell their obesity patients that the LAP-BAND is a gimmick, nothing but a modified 'Angelchik.'

This can't be any further from the truth. Most of the surgeons making this statement have never even seen an Angelchik prosthesis, let alone have any experience with one. Furthermore, the LAP-BAND is anything but a gimmick. It is a wonderfully simple tool, or aid, in weight reduction. It is somewhat simpler to perform than a Gastric Bypass procedure and certainly has a lower risk of leakage and complications. The argument has been made that a bypass procedure is safer than a LAP-BAND after the initial two weeks, if the patient does not have a leak. This is not exactly true. When all bypass patients are examined after 4 to 5 years, what is the gastro-gastric fistulization rate?

Does this matter?

American surgeons have not been exactly honest intellectually with many patients. We need to do a better job with this simple fact. We need to tell patients the whole truth about all procedures when asked. I was an obese surgeon. My BMI was 44. I now have a BMI of 25. I had a LAP-BAND one year ago. I reached my goal weight after 10 months. I needed to lose over 100 pounds of weight. I personally perform LAP-BAND surgery. The huge majority of my patients have not done as well as I have.

Why not?

Are they not as motivated as I have been?

The probable answer lies in the need for any surgical procedure. When the patient has had many successful attempts over long periods of time at losing weight, they tend to be the most successful.

Have I set the bar too high?

Probably so. Patients now routinely call our coordinator demanding to know why they are not doing as well as others, especially their surgeon. It pays to have a coordinator who is also a LAP-BAND patient who can explain what the process is truly like."

Lee Grossbard, M.D.

I Was Truly Suffering
by
Lisa Geraci-Ruppert

"My name is Lisa Geraci-Ruppert and I'm 33 years old. When I reached my maximum weight that caused me heart ache, I topped the scales at 232 pounds; that was heavy for a person measuring 5'3". My parents were morbidly obese, and my father died from it and heart disease at 51. When I started with Dr. Gabriel and LI Bariatric Center, I was suffering from multiple injuries that had greatly reduced my mobility. It didn't help that I was gulping 2 liters of soda a day; but even so, I was normally eating only one large meal a day. I had gained so much weight that I could barely function. I was taking shots for pain regularly in my feet for heel spurs and bunions. I was borderline for knee replacements, both of them. My life was revolving around what doctor I had to see next. I was going down hill fast.

I spoke with Dr. Gabriel on the phone and we discussed the surgery before I went to the Center. He put my mind at ease with all the information he gave me. I took the tests that the LI Bariatric Center sent me to have and they discovered that I had very high triglycerides and cholesterol levels, a fatty liver, and gallstones. LI Bariatric Center got me approved for my surgery and I was well on my way to recovery.

On August 7, 2002, I had my LAP-BAND surgically placed and my gallbladder removed. Dr. Gabriel really didn't want to do both at the same time, but I wanted to get it over with and I am so glad that he did it for me. I had extra pain, but all in all, I began to lose weight right away instead of waiting for a second surgery. I had retained water in the hospital from the IV. It took me about a month and some water pills to get back on track, but it has been a breeze since. I have minimal scares and they are fading. I started the Optifast™ shakes a little earlier than what was required, so I lost approximately 14 pounds before my surgery. I still use them occasionally as a supplement for breakfast or lunch on the run, and they have also helped with the great results that I have made.

Well, now I am 125 pounds and maintaining. I have my life back and I feel great. The pain from my prior injuries has been reduced. All my blood levels have gone down and my health has been great. I am down to a size 5 and it feels so wonderful to be slim. No one believes me when they see my before pictures. I feel and look like a new person thanks to this incredible device. I'm in debt to my awesome surgeon and the support and diligence of LI Bariatric Center.

As a personal note here, I want to thank you, Dr. Gabriel, for all of your good humor, great bedside manner, and encouragement throughout every step of the way. It is wonderful to have a doctor so interested in your well-being and one that you can talk to like a real person and not just a caregiver. I feel very lucky to have had you as my surgeon. I hope I have made you proud of your excellent work.

To Dory Ferraro, your Bariatric Center has been a wonderful experience for me. From my first day, I felt accepted and understood. Your advice and guidance has helped to keep me focused and encouraged, and your diligence in getting me approved so quickly was amazing. Thank you for bearing with all my stupid questions and with great humor. You are both outstanding professionals and I am honored to have had the opportunity to work with you to achieve my goal of a healthy life."

Lisa Geraci-Ruppert
North Baldwin, NY

I Lost 200 Pounds
by
Rick Rush

"I woke up more tired than when I went to bed. I caught myself gasping for air several times during the night. My heart was racing and I knew that losing weight was no longer an option, but rather a necessity. I was fully aware that when you are 5'9" and weigh 395 pounds, your future is tenuous at best.

I had had high blood pressure for years and my knees were killing me. I needed to do something to resolve these issues. I had engaged in numerous diet and exercise plans throughout my life and had lost weight, but I was never able to keep it off. I was always hungry and knew that I could not control my food intake over an extended period of time. Therefore, I began to eagerly surf the Web for information on weight-loss surgery.

I discovered the LAP-BAND and educated myself by reading thousands of messages on various boards. In my case, insurance would not cover LAP-BAND surgery, so money was an issue, but quality medical care was my primary concern.

My research led me to conclude that the LAP-BAND weight-loss surgery was for me. The LAP-BAND controls how much you eat. It does this without touching your intestinal system like the Gastric Bypass does. I chose the LAP-BAND because it was the least invasive weight-loss surgery and it had the lowest complication rate.

I chose Dr. Ortiz for my surgery, foremost for his expertise and his experience with the LAP-BAND. I was impressed with the fact that he was currently training American surgeons on the LAP-BAND and the fact that he had installed more than a thousand bands over a seven-year period.

I contacted his patient coordinator and scheduled surgery within two weeks. I immediately got in to see my internist and had an EKG and blood work, because I didn't want to travel 3,000 miles only to discover that I wasn't a good candidate for surgery. My internist was from Peru and had seen many successful band surgeries in Central America, so he was very excited for me and encouraged me to have the surgery. My blood pressure was 165/130 and my sugar level was 116. He told me that I was borderline diabetic, and he gave me literature on sugar diabetes. He also told me that I had sleep apnea.

I flew in to San Diego and took a taxi to Dr. Ortiz's office. I went through a series of pre-surgery tests and nothing precluded me from having the surgery. I had been on a high-protein liquid diet for 10 days, so I had lost 15 pounds, but I was starving. Surgery was scheduled for the next morning. I had had surgery twice before in the United States, but this was different. I was so impressed to meet the whole surgical team. I never met a surgical assistant or an anesthesiologist with my prior surgeries.

The surgery took place at a very modern facility. The hospital room had a hospital bed and a full-sized bed. I made the trip by myself, but the rooms are designed for a 'significant other' to be able to stay with you. The surgery went very smoothly and took all of 25 minutes to complete. I stayed in the hospital two nights. My recovery was quick. I experienced some discomfort and mild pain, but no significant pain.

The first two weeks after surgery were amazing. I lost 25 pounds and my knees felt great. The most incredible thing, however, was the total absence of hunger. I never in my life experienced this feeling of control. I was no longer controlled by the desire for food. I ate nothing but a little chicken broth for two weeks and felt totally satisfied. I knew in just a couple of days after surgery that if my appetite was going to stay in check for the long run, that I had just the tool I needed in the LAP-BAND to control my destiny.

I lost 100 pounds in the first eight months. I got four fills and my appetite was in check. I consumed about 60 grams of protein and 1,300 calories a day. I drank about 4 liters of water a day. The weight went flying off and my health issues resolved themselves. My blood pressure is now under 110/75, and my sugar is now in the low end of the normal range at 84. I no longer have sleep apnea.

I started to walk five and a half miles per day after month 8 because I felt I wanted to get more fit. Walking has helped me get stronger and improve my muscle tone. As each month goes by and the weight comes off, I become more determined than ever to reach my goal weight. I am now 12 months post surgery, and I have lost 205 pounds. I have recently started a weight-lifting program, and I am determined to get down to 170 pounds.

I am very thankful that I found Dr. Ortiz and the LAP-BAND. The LAP-BAND has been the answer for me."
Rick Rush

Isn't it wonderful that we live in an age of high-tech medicine? What will the future bring for the obese? Until then, we have the band—the wonderful LAP-BAND—in all its useful ways. Try it. It's the safest way to surgical weight-loss. I know, I have performed all the variations of weight-loss surgery and the LAP-BAND is the safest, most effective weight-control surgery in the world.

PERSONAL MEDICAL LOG

THIS INITIAL INFORMATION CAN HELP YOU GO THROUGH YOUR INITIAL CONSULTATION AND KEEP TRACK OF YOUR MEDICAL HISTORY.

PERSONAL INFORMATION

NAME_____ DATE_____

DATE OF BIRTH_____ AGE____ GENDER ☐ M ☐ F

E-MAIL Address _____

How long have you been considering weight-loss surgery?_____

Have you done any research regarding weight-loss Surgery? ☐ Yes ☐ No

If yes, what type?_____

How did you hear about this program?_____

Do you have a friend or family member who has had weight

loss surgery? ☐ Yes ☐ No If yes, who?_____

WEIGHT AND WEIGHT-LOSS HISTORY:

Age you were first overweight:_____ Highest weight:_____ When:_____

Age you first started dieting:___ Weight range last 5 years: _____ to _____

Approximate weight at age 18:_____

Method of Weight-loss	Yes	No	Date(s) Attempted	Duration of Effort	Maximum Loss
Jenny Craig					
Nutri-Systems					
Weight Watchers					
Opti-fast Medi Fast					
O.A. ot TOPS					
Fen/Phen Redux					
Meridia					
Xenical					
Over-the-counter diet aids					
Atkins Diet					
Other:					
Other:					

Which method of weight-loss did you prefer? Why? _____

_____

What is the most challenging part of trying to lose weight? _____

_____

YOUR LIFESTYLE

DIET: Please circle the best answer for each question:

1) How often do you eat three meals in a day (breakfast, lunch, and dinner)?
   a. Always   c. Some days
   b. Most days   d. Rarely or never

2) Which meal is most often skipped?
   a. Breakfast   c. Dinner
   b. Lunch   d. None skipped usually

3) How often do you "snack" (defined as any food eaten between meals or after dinner)?
   a) Rarely or never   c. 2–3 times/day
   b) 1 time/day   d. Often graze on food throughout the day

4) Foods commonly eaten between meals or after dinner:

_____

5) How often do you eat sweets (candy, donuts, pastries, etc.)?
   a. < 3 times/week   c. 1 time/day
   b. 3–5 times/week   d. 2 or more times/day

6) How frequently do you eat until very full or uncomfortable?
   a. Most meals   c. Occasionally
   b. Often   d. Rarely or never

7) My usual beverages consist of (check all that apply):
   ____ Water   Amount/day _____
   ____ Coffee   Amount/day _____
   ____ Juice   Amount/day _____
   ____ Regular soda   Amount/day _____
   ____ Diet soda/carbonated waters   Amount/day _____

_____ Diet non-carbonated drinks   Amount/day _____
_____ Alcohol   Amount/day _____

8) How often do you typically eat in restaurants? Count breakfasts,
   lunches, & dinners (do not include fast food/take-out food):
   a. 1 time/week or less
   b. 2–3 times/week
   c. 4 times/week or more

9) How often do you eat fast food or take-out meals? Count all breakfasts, lunches, and dinners:
   a. 1 time/week or less
   b. 2–3 times/week
   c. 4 times/week or more

10) What is your usual fruit and vegetable intake (combined)?
    a. < 1 serving/day   c. 3–4 servings/day
    b. 1–2 servings/day   d. 5 or more servings/day

11) List examples of typical high protein foods eaten:
    a. _____   b. _____

12) How long does it usually take you to eat a meal?
    a. 1–10 minutes   c. 20–30 minutes
    b. 10–20 minutes   d. at least 30 minutes

PHYSICAL EXERCISE

At the present time, are you a regular exerciser? _____

Do you have any physical restrictions that keep you from exercising?
☐ Yes ☐ No Explain _____

What form(s) of exercise (walking, swimming, etc.)? _____
_____

How many days per week do you exercise? _____

How long does each session last? _____ minutes

MEDICATIONS

Prescription Medications	Dose	Frequency
Non-Prescription Medications	Dose	Frequency

SURGERIES

Date	Surgery

HOSPITALIZATION

Date	Illness	Treatment

Are you allergic to any medications? _____

Are you allergic to surgical tape? ☐ Yes ☐ No   Latex? ☐ Yes ☐ No

Iodine? ☐ Yes ☐ No Other allergies: _____

MEDICAL HISTORY

Cardiovascular	Current	Past	Don't	Gastrointestinal	Current	Past	Don't
High Blood				Heartburn			
Irregular Heart Beat				Reflux Disease			
Stroke				Hiatal Hernia			
Heart Attack				Gastric Ulcer			
Echocardio-gram or				Irritable Bowel Syndrome			
Blood Clots in Lungs				Diverticulitis			
Swelling in				Ulcerative Colitis			
Elevated				Crohns Disease			
Heart Surgery				Gynecological			
Respiratory				Last Menstrual Period:			
Asthma				Number of Pregnancies:			
Shortness of Breath @				Number of Births:			
Shortness of Breath with				Date of Last Mammogram:			
Bronchitis				Date of Last Pap Smear:			
Need Oxygen Therapy				Hormone			
Pneumonia				Birth Control			
Sleep Apnea				Urinary			
Do you use a				Difficulty with Urination			
Endocrine				Frequent Bladder Infections			
Type 2 Diabetes				Urinary Stress Incontinence			
Blood Sugar Range:				Kidney Infection			
Pre Diabetes				Musculoskeletal			
Complica-tions of				Back Pain			
Polycystic Ovarian				Hip Pain			
Thyroid Disease				Knee Pain			
Psychological				Ankle/Foot Pain			

Cardiovascular	Current	Past	Don't	Gastrointestinal	Current	Past	Don't
Depression				Osteoarthritis			
Panic Attacks				Plantar Fasciitis			
Anxiety				Hematological			
Bi-polar Disease				Anemia			
Eating Disorder				AIDS/HIV			
Obsessive Compulsive				Blood Transfusion			
Special Needs:				Bleeding Disorder			
Mobility Issues				Other Conditions			
Hearing Impaired				Cancer:			
Vision Impaired				Other:			
English Interpreter				Other:			

FAMILY HISTORY:

Marital Status: ☐ Single ☐ Married ☐ Divorced ☐ Widowed

Gender: ☐ Male ☐ Female

Occupation: _____

How many hours a week do you work? _____

Number of children _____ Ages of Children _____

Do you care for elder relatives? _____ Who? _____

What is your involvement in their care? _____

_____

With whom do you reside? _____

Is there obesity in the family? ☐ Yes ☐ No If yes, who? _____

Medical Illness in the family: ☐ Yes ☐ No If so, what?

☐ Clotting Disorders ☐ Coronary Artery Disease ☐ Diabetes

☐ Hypertension ☐ Cancer ☐ Other _____

Have you ever smoked cigarettes/cigars? ☐ Yes ☐ No

Do you smoke now? ☐ Yes ☐ No

When did you quit? _____

How much did you smoke per day? _____

Do you drink alcohol? ☐ Yes ☐ No

What type of alcohol do you consume? _____

Number of drinks per week _____ (Note: 1 drink = 12oz. beer or 5 oz. wine or 1.5 oz. hard liquor/distilled spirits.)

Have you or are you currently using any recreational/illegal drugs?

☐ Yes ☐ No Explain: _____

Have you ever been a binge eater? ☐ Yes ☐ No

Are you now? ☐ Yes ☐ No Frequency of binges:_____

Have you ever purged (induced vomiting) after eating too much?

☐ Yes ☐ No Do you now? ☐ Yes ☐ No

Do you have a history of abuse? (Please include emotional, physical, mental, substance, or other types of abuse issues you have dealt with. This information is **extremely** important and very confidential. Honesty is needed in order to provide you with the best possible treatment plan.)

_____

_____

_____

Have you ever been in treatment with:

Psychologist? (therapist) ☐ Yes ☐ No

Psychiatrist? ☐ Yes ☐ No

One-on-one counseling or group sessions? _____

For how long? _____

Name of psychologist or psychiatrist _____

Have you ever been hospitalized for mental health reasons?

☐ Yes ☐ No Explain: _____

_____

Have you ever been treated for alcohol abuse or chemical dependency?

Explain: _____

_____

Have you ever attended AA or NA meetings? ☐ Yes ☐ No

Explain your present life stressors: _____

_____

Explain the present support system you rely upon (church, spouse, family, friends, coworkers, etc.): _____

_____

What are your goals for weight-loss with LAP-BAND surgery?

_____

_____

What concerns or fears do you have? _____
_____

PHYSICIANS: (Please Complete)

Specialty	Name	Address	Phone and Fax
Primary Care			
OBGYN			
Orthopedic			
Endocrinologist			
Psychologist/			
Chiropractor			
Other			

FOOD:

A 4-day food log can be used before a fill or when a patient has trouble with the band. It should always be shown to the treating doctor.

4-day Food Log

Date/Time	Food/Drink Consumed	Amount	Where did you eat?	Degree of Hunger 1 (not) – 10 (very)	Degree of Fullness 1 (not) – 10 (very)

MY LAP-BAND JOURNAL

Sample Weight-Loss Log

Date	Weight
7/25 (Preop)	297
8/3	283
8/10	279
8/17	276.5
8/24	273
8/31	273
9/7	268
9/14	269
9/21	267
9/28	267
10/5	264
10/12	263
10/19	263
10/25	255
11/2	258
11/9	258
11/16	257
11/23	255

My Weight-Loss Log

Date	Weight

Internet Resources and Links

There are a large number of sources on the Internet of information on LAP-BAND surgery and on other types of weight-loss surgery.

OFFICIAL LAP-BAND SITES
There are only two web sites in America that are the official sites for INAMED Health, manufacturer of the LAP-BAND implant

For the United States it is:
http://www.INAMED.com

For Latin America it is:
www.mecachrome-medical.com.

These websites offer information for patients on their products and are especially valuable because they list the surgeons that have undergone the training in this technique.

OFFICIAL SITE ON WEIGHTLOSS SURGERY
http://www.wlsinfo.org.uk/ British Guide to Weight-Loss Surgery

http://www.weightlosssurgeryinfo.com/pages/what_is/index.jsp General informative site, not leaning toward any procedure.

http://bariatricsearch.com/ Directs patients to surgeons performing various types of weight-loss surgery. Features a map of the United States, and you click on a state to get information and links. May be sponsored (where the doctor or clinic pays for the referral).

http://www.asbs.org/ Website of the American Society for Bariatric Surgery. Features phone numbers of members and a few useful links.

http://www.smco.org.mx/obesity3/ingles/mensaje.asp Site of the Mexican Society of Obesity Surgery. Dr. Ortiz was the President of MSOS in 2002–2003.

http://www.sages.org/sg_pub30.html Society of American Gastrointestinal Endoscopic Surgeons article on "Guidelines for Laparoscopic and Conventional Surgical Treatment of Morbid Obesity."

http://www.cdc.gov/nccdphp/dnpa/obesity/index.htm Center for Disease Control site dealing with Obesity.

http://www.sls.org/ Society of Laparoscopic Surgeons home site. Includes surgeon locator not specific to LAP-BANDs

http://www.cjmedical.com/pdfs/AGB350.PDF Soft band information from its manufacturer.

http://www.asbs.org/html/story/chapter1.html "The Story of Surgery for Obesity" by Dr. Alex MacGregor FACS, part of the site of the American Society for Bariatric Surgery. A bit technical, but interesting.

http://www.obesity.org/ American Obesity Association

LEGAL AND INSURANCE ISSUES
http://www.weightforlife.com ® has over 12 years of extensive experience in working with insurance companies nationwide in acquiring preauthorization and fighting appeals

http://www.obesitylaw.com/ Walter Lindstrom is an attorney renowned for help in getting insurers to cover LAP-BAND surgery.

FOOD AND NUTRITION SITES
http://www.meals.com/ Yummy recipes with nutritional info.

http://www.new-fitness.com/nutrition/protein.html Guide to keeping your protein intake at proper levels.

http://www.recipe4living.com/recipes_4-18.html Healthy recipes

http://store.yahoo.com/cntr4weightloss/catalog.html High-protein and other weight-loss products catalog

http://www.ntwrks.com/~mikev/chart3a.htm Calorie, Fat, and Protein chart for a wide range of food.

http://www.room42.com/nutrition/basal.shtml Basal metabolism calculator.

http://www.unjury.com/ Protein supplement source.

http://www.veryfine.com/ Healthy products.

SUPPORT GROUPS
Listed below are a wide variety of Internet groups, where people of all experience levels ask questions, give advice, relate their experiences, and in general try to help.
http://www.lapbandforum.com
http://www.wlssuccess.com/lapbanders.htm

http://www.spotlighthealth.com/common/SG/topics.asp?m=1&sb=25

http://www.lapbandtalk.com

http://www.obesityhelp.com

BMI Calculator*

5'0" - 6'4" — 165 - 300 Pounds

Weight in pounds	165	170	175	180	185	190	195	200	205	210	215	220	225	230	240	250	260	270	280	290	300
Height																					
5'0"	32	33	34	35	36	37	38	39	40	41	42	43	44	45	46	48	50	52	54	56	58
5'1"	31	32	33	34	35	36	36	37	38	39	40	41	42	43	45	47	49	51	53	54	58
5'2"	30	31	32	33	33	34	35	36	37	38	39	40	41	42	44	46	48	49	51	53	55
5'3"	29	30	31	32	32	33	34	35	36	37	38	39	40	41	42	44	46	48	49	51	53
5'4"	28	29	30	31	31	32	33	34	35	36	37	38	39	40	41	43	44	46	48	50	51
5'5"	27	28	29	30	30	31	32	33	34	35	35	36	37	38	40	42	43	45	46	48	50
5'6"	26	27	28	29	29	30	31	32	33	34	34	35	36	37	38	40	42	43	45	47	48
5'7"	25	26	27	28	29	29	30	31	32	33	33	34	35	36	37	39	41	42	44	45	47
5'8"	25	25	26	27	28	28	29	30	31	32	32	33	34	35	36	38	39	41	42	44	45
5'9"	24	25	25	26	27	28	28	29	30	31	31	32	33	34	35	37	38	40	41	43	44
5'10"	23	24	25	25	26	27	28	28	29	30	30	31	32	33	34	36	37	39	40	42	43
5'11"	23	23	24	25	25	26	27	28	28	29	30	31	32	33	34	35	36	38	39	40	42
6'0"	22	23	23	24	25	25	26	27	27	28	29	30	30	31	32	34	35	36	38	39	40
6'1"	21	22	23	23	24	25	25	26	27	27	28	29	30	31	32	33	34	35	37	38	39
6'2"	21	21	22	23	23	24	25	25	26	27	27	28	29	30	31	32	33	34	36	37	38
6'3"	20	21	22	22	23	24	24	25	25	26	27	27	28	29	30	31	32	33	35	36	37
6'4"	20	21	21	22	22	23	23	24	25	25	26	26	27	28	29	30	31	32	33	34	36

All BMI numbers are rounded off. For a more detailed calculator, go to web site:

www.halls.md/body-mass-index/bmi.htm

Glossary of Terms

Adjustability. The feature of a band that allows it to be tightened or loosened.

Adjustable Gastric Banding (LAP-BAND). Placement of an adjustable silicone band around the stomach to restrict food intake.

Adjustment. Another name for a fill or an unfill, where the amount of saline solution in the band is increased or decreased to control the size of the stoma.

AGB. Adjustable Gastric Banding

Angelchik. An anti gastro-esophageal reflux procedure, in which a ring-shaped radiopaque prosthesis is placed around the esophagus after reduction of a hiatal hernia, usually below the diaphragm.

Balloon. (Gastric Balloon). With this procedure, a device much like a balloon is implanted in the stomach and then inflated. It takes up space in the stomach so that less food can be ingested.

Bandster. 1. Common term for someone who has had a band operation. Not all banded people are necessarily Bandsters. 2. Member of an online, local, and national group which share the Bandster name.

Bariatrics. The branch of medicine that deals with the treatment of obesity. From the Greek *barys,* meaning heavy and -*iatrics*, meaning medical treatment.

Bash. 1. A Bandster convention (The Tijuana Bandster Bash was the first.) 2. To denigrate a particular doctor (considered poor form).

Biliopancreatic Diversion. A discontinued weight-loss surgery method developed in 1970s, in which less of the small intestine was bypassed, reducing kidney and liver difficulties.

Biliopancreatic Diversion with Duodenal Switch. An improvement over the biliopancreatic diversion, increasing the amount of the small intestine left intact and not removing the pyloric valve that connects the stomach to the small intestine. This began in the early 1990s.

BioEnterics. The former name of INAMED Corporation, Cf. INAMED.

BMI. Body Mass Index

Body Mass Index. It is the person's weight in kilograms divided by the square of their height in meters. A table in Appendix 3 offers a quick way to calculate your BMI. It is an excellent measuring tool for just about everyone except extremely muscular people such as bodybuilders. A person with a BMI of 25 or more is considered overweight. Obesity is defined as a BMI of 30 to 40. More than 40 is considered morbidly obese.

Co-morbidity. Presence of a second disease or condition influencing the care or treatment of a patient, and which in the hospital setting is expected to increase the length of stay by at least one day for most patients.

Coordinator. Since there are so many questions asked by people considering LAP-BAND surgery, it is common for the surgeons who perform it to have a Coordinator who answers the questions and arranges the surgeries and fill appointments. Many also handle hotel reservations and shuttle service for patients who must travel to the surgeon's location.

Co-payment. This is an amount that an insured person pays for medical services at the time of the procedure. For gastrointestinal surgery, co-payment is typically 20–30% of the amount billed. Note that insurers only pay a relatively small percentage of the amount billed.

Detachment of the Port. Disconnection of the hose connecting the port to the LAP-BAND. Not uncommon in bands until 2001. Newer models have effectively eliminated this problem.

Dumping. LAP-BAND patients do not experience dumping, but it is a huge problem for Gastric Bypass (Roux-en-Y) patients. The small intestine cannot handle concentrated calories. If the patient consumes foods that contains sugar or fat (ice cream or M&M's are the classic examples), this segment of intestine reacts by creating the dumping syndrome. It is characterized by palpitations (fast heart rate), a clammy feeling, queasiness, and nausea, sometimes vomiting, and sometimes diarrhea. Usually, the patient feels weak and must lie down for thirty to sixty minutes. The dumping syndrome is not dangerous but it feels absolutely horrible.

Emotional Eating. Eating in response to feelings instead of hunger. The feelings that cause most emotional eating are anger, hopelessness, feeling of lack of control, feeling unappreciated, and boredom.

Erosion. A complication where the band abrades the stomach. If untreated, it may eventually result in puncture of the stomach. Uncommon.

Excess weight. The weight in excess that would put the LAP-BAND patient at a BMI of 25.

FAQ. Frequently Asked Questions. A typical feature of websites about new technologies, they are the questions that come up again and again, so they are collected in one place for pre-LAP-BAND patients to refer to before asking a question that has been answered many times.

Fill. Injection of saline solution through the port to inflate the band to tighten the band around the stomach, thus decreasing the size of the stoma.

Fluoroscope. A real-time X-ray machine that makes it possible to see internal organs in motion. It shows the internal organs on a TV monitor and is used in fills (adjustments) with a barium solution, which shows up clearly on the fluoroscope, to show how much fluid passes through the stoma.

Fobi Pouch Gastric Bypass. Dr. Mal Fobi of Hawaiian Gardens, California, has been performing an operation creating the Fobi Limiting Proximal Gastric Pouch, which consists of a pouch smaller than 30 cc with a 5.5–6.5 cm long nonadjustable band around the stomach. The end of the pouch is attached to the small intestine.

Gastric Balloon (Gastric Bubble). With this procedure, a device much like a balloon is implanted in the stomach and then inflated. It takes up space in the stomach so that less food can be ingested. This is a temporary stopgap measure for those with BMI over 55.

Gastric Bypass. Also known as Stomach Stapling, Roux-en-Y, and RNY.

Gastroplasty. The basic stomach-stapling surgery, which worked on restriction only. Abandoned, because the pouch and stoma enlarged over time, and the patient gained back the excess weight.

GERD. Gastro-Esophageal Reflux Disease. A disorder in which there is recurrent return of stomach contents back up into the esophagus, frequently causing heartburn, a symptom of irritation of the esophagus by stomach acid. This can lead to scarring and stricture of the esophagus, which can require stretching (dilating). 10% of patients with GERD develop Barrett's esophagus, which increases the risk of cancer of the esophagus. 80% of patients with GERD also have a hiatal hernia.

Goal Weight. The target a LAP-BAND patient sets in terms of the desired weight.

Hiatal hernia. The abnormal protrusion of the lower esophagus and/or portion of the stomach through the eso-phageal hiatus or the opening in the diaphragm. Surgeons must repair this before a band can be placed.

INAMED. A corporation based in Santa Barbara, California, that produces the LAP-BAND ® in addition to other medical products, including a new silicone breast implant. (See Appendix 2 for links to its website.)

Jejuno-Ileal Bypass (JIB). Obsolete weight-loss surgery performed in the 1950s and 1960s.

Joule. The term used in Australia for what is called a calorie in the United States and a kilocalorie in other parts of the world.

LAP-BAND. Shorthand for the INAMED BioEnterics LAP-BAND System® aka Adjustable Gastric Banding Placement of an adjustable silicone band around the stomach to restrict food intake.

Laparoscopic Gastric Bypass. Laparoscopic version of the Gastric Bypass, cf.

Laparoscopy. The insertion of a thin, lighted tube (called a laparoscope) through the abdominal wall to inspect the inside of the abdomen for the purpose of diagnosis, biopsy, or surgery. It is a type of endoscope but with a tiny video camera.

Liquids. While the dictionary may have a different definition, for the freshly banded person the definition of a liquid is whatever can be sucked through a straw. In the first four to seven days after surgery, the newly banded person should only drink clear liquids, ones that are translucent. In the next four to seven days, the newly banded person can drink any liquid.

After the one-month postoperative period, banded people will find that liquid meals such as protein shakes and supplement drinks such as Ensure should be avoided, as they do not fill the pouch long enough to trigger the feeling of fullness that is important to the success of the band. Additionally, banded people should avoid ingesting liquids from twenty minutes before to one hour after a meal of solid food. (Some surgeons recommend even longer periods of abstaining from liquids.)

Lurker. Someone who reads the postings on the various groups but contributes rarely or never.

Malabsorption. One of the two ways that surgery causes weight-loss, by removing or bypassing a part of the small intestines so there is less intestinal area to absorb food ingested. Cf Restriction. Causes loose, smelly feces, flatulence; need to use vitamin supplements.

MIDBand. An adjustable gastric band produced by Médical Innovation Développement of Villeurbanne, France. It does not have a rigid frame, as does the INAMED LAP-BAND. Not approved in the United States.

Newbie. Term used in the groups for a newly banded person who is going through early phases of learning how to live with the band and get results.

Obesity. Doctors use body mass index, or BMI, as a measure of obesity. It is the person's weight in kilograms divided by the square of their height in meters. A table in Appendix 3 offers a quick way to calculate your BMI. It is an excellent measuring tool for just about everyone except extremely muscular people such as bodybuilders. A person with a BMI of 25 or more is considered overweight. Obesity is defined as a BMI of 30 to 40. Over 40 is considered morbidly obese.

Band (Swedish Band, SAGB®). An adjustable gastric band produced Atos Medical of Sweden under license by Obtech of Switzerland. As of this writing, it is in the testing phase for introduction by US giant Johnson.

Obtech & Johnson®. A band not approved in the United States.

PB. Productive Burp. Not really a burp, but a regurgitation of some of the contents of the pouch that occurs when the LAP-BAND patient has not chewed thoroughly enough, and a piece of food has clogged the stoma.

Port. 1. The reservoir for saline solution connected to the LAP-BAND by a small hose. (See also Disconnection of the port.) 2. The entry incision for laparoscopic surgery.

Pouch. The upper part of the stomach of a LAP-BAND patient, generally about the size of a wine glass. Connected to the rest of the stomach through the Stoma cf.

Pre-Bandster. Term used on Bandster groups and organizations to denote someone considering LAP-BAND surgery or who has scheduled it.

Pulmonologist. A physician specializing in lung diseases and breathing problems.

Restriction. One of the two ways that surgery causes weight-loss, is by restricting the amount of food that can be ingested at any one time. Cf. Malabsorption.

RNY. Also known as Gastric Bypass, Stomach Stapling, and Roux-en-Y.

Roux-en-Y. Also known as Gastric Bypass, Stomach Stapling, and RNY.

Sabotage. Actions, often unthinking and unintentional, of spouses, children, friends, and colleagues, that tend to divert the LAP-BAND patient from following the regimen which will result in weight-loss. Also, the LAP-BAND patient can fall into old patterns and sabotage the patient.

SAGB. Swedish Adjustable Gastric Band (Swedish Band or Obtech Band.) Not approved in the United States.

Self-pay. When insurance providers, HMOS, and PPOs refuse to cover LAP-BAND surgery, the patient pays for the operation out of pocket.

Slime. A very viscous form of saliva created in profusion when a LAP-BAND patient has swallowed a morsel of food too large for the stoma and which has blocked the stoma. Cf PB, which is the following step.

Slippage. Movement of the band on the stomach away from its original position, generally toward the esophagus. Prevented with skilled surgical techniques.

Stoma. The hole between the top and bottom parts of the stomach. Think of it as the narrow part of an hourglass.

Stomach Stapling. Also known as Gastric Bypass, Roux-en-Y, and RNY.

Swedish Band. An adjustable gastric band produced by Atos Medical of Sweden under license from Obtech of Switzerland and currently in the testing phase for introduction by US giant Johnson & Johnson. Not approved in the United States.

Sweet spot. The fill level that is the ideal balance between being too tight and too loose, where the weight just seems to melt off.

Unfill. Removal of saline solution through the port to deflate the band and relax the band around the stomach, thus increasing the size of the stoma. Used in case of illness, pregnancy, or attaining goal weight. CF fill.

Vertical Banded Gastroplasty. A surgery which uses a non-adjustable band. Largely abandoned because the pouch and stoma enlarged over time, and the patient gained back the excess weight.

About the Author

Ariel Alfonso Alfredo Ortiz Lagardère, M.D FACS

Dr. Ortiz has done numerous surgical procedures (mainly Lap Bands) on grateful patients. He is not only a leader in this growing medical field of LAP-BAND Surgery that offers sound weight-loss control, but in addition, he has the honor of having trained many surgeons in the United States and other countries in the procedure, both as a proctor for the makers of the LAP-BAND, INAMED Corp, located in Santa Barbara, California and in his own clinic..

He is among those highly qualified surgeons who have contributed to the on-going fight against obesity with a large contingent of patients who are thinner due to his efforts of placing a LAP-BAND.

In the field of medicine and surgery, Dr. Ortiz has an outstanding resume. He is a member of laparoscopy societies in Mexico and the United State with these credentials: a Fellow of the *American College of Surgeons* and a full member of the *American Society of Bariatric Surgery*, the *International Federation for Surgery of Obesity,* and Professor of Surgery and Director of *Minimally Invasive Surgery Institute of NW Mexico.*

Dr. Ortiz has lectured extensively around the world and is frequently designated as keynote speaker at weight-loss and bariatric events. As a researcher in the field of weight-loss surgery, he is active in research and development in laparoscopic surgery. In the past decade he has hosted numerous workshops where dozens of surgeons from a number of countries have attended these workshops to learn the technique of LAP-BAND surgery. In addition, he is one of the leading surgeons in laparoscopic hernia repair.

Without reservation, it can be said that Dr. Ortiz is among the leading LAP-BAND surgeons of the world.

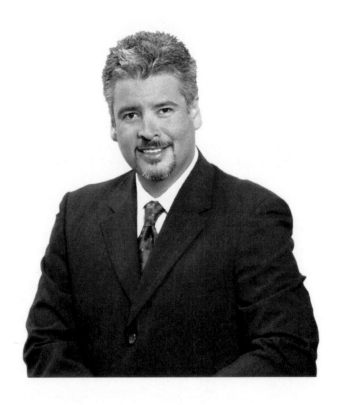